BREAST CANCER DIAGNOSIS

BREAST CANCER DIAGNOSIS

Gerald S. Johnston and A. Eric Jones
Department of Nuclear Medicine, Clinical Center
National Institutes of Health

PLENUM MEDICAL BOOK COMPANY • New York and London

Library of Congress Cataloging in Publication Data

Main entry under title:

Breast cancer diagnosis.

Includes bibliographical references and index.
1. Breast–Cancer–Diagnosis. 2. Radioisotope scanning. I. Johnston, Gerald S., 1930- II. Jones, Alfred Eric, 1935- [DNLM: 1. Breast neoplasms–Diagnosis. 2. Radioisotope scanning. 3. Mammography. WP870 B826]
RC280.B8B68 616.9'94'49 75-31980
ISBN 978-1-4684-2219-1 ISBN 978-1-4684-2217-7 (eBook)
DOI 10.1007/978-1-4684-2217-7

Plenum Publishing Corporation
227 West 17th Street, New York, N. Y. 10011

United Kingdom edition published by Plenum Publishing Company, Ltd.
Davis House (4th Floor), 8 Scrubs Lane, Harlesden, London, NW10 6SE, England

Plenum Medical Book Company is an imprint of Plenum Publishing Corporation

Softcover reprint of the hardcover 1st edition 1975

CONTRIBUTORS

National Institutes of Health, Bethesda, Maryland

George S. Flinn, M.D.
Department of Radiology, Clinical Center

Robert S. Frankel, M.D.
Department of Nuclear Medicine, Clinical Center

Robert S. Francis, M.D.
Department of Radiology, Clinical Center

Gerald S. Johnston, M.D.
Department of Nuclear Medicine, Clinical Center

Alfred E. Jones, M.D.
Department of Nuclear Medicine, Clinical Center

James N. Ingle, M.D.
Medical Oncology, Medicine Branch
National Cancer Institute

Stanley M. Levenson, M.D.
Department of Nuclear Medicine, Clinical Center

Steven D. Richman, M.D.
Department of Nuclear Medicine, Clinical Center

Douglass C. Tormey, M.D., Ph.D.
Medical Oncology, Medicine Branch,
National Cancer Institute

PREFACE

Breast carcinoma is a dreaded disease. The incidence of breast cancer, which appears to be increasing, is 1 in 1500 women with an annual death rate of 4,000 from this disease in the United States (1). It is a cancer which threatens its victims with mutilation as well as early death. Although response to therapy has not been good, improved methods for earlier and more complete diagnosis are providing hope for better results.

When a woman presents herself for routine breast examination, what diagnostic procedures are indicated? If a breast mass is present, what diagnostic and therapeutic methods are employed? When the mass proves to be malignant, what then? Should biopsy and mastectomy be a combined procedure? Should a positive biopsy be followed by a complete diagnostic work-up before definitive therapy is undertaken? While some answers may seem obvious and others less obvious, common medical practices vary considerably in response to all of these situations. No easy formula exists. Each patient must be given individual consideration and her* treatment carefully planned to incorporate all the diagnostic findings. Experience to date indicates that some diagnostic and therapeutic procedures have established efficacy while others are not very helpful and still others need more evaluation before their usefulness can be assessed fully.

Traditionally, treatment of breast cancer has been surgical. Through the years poor results from surgery, along with acquisition of knowledge of the lymphatic spread of this malignancy, prompted more and more extensive surgical procedures. In the 1890's Halsted developed the radical mastectomy which then became a main surgical treatment for breast cancer (2). The 1940's saw the introduction of both radiation therapy and hormonal manipulations as therapeutic augmentations to surgery. Chemotherapy was added in the 1960's and continues to be developed in the 1970's. More conservative surgical modifications away from the Halsted procedure have been coming into vogue, and the place of radiation therapy in association with surgery continues to be investigated. Since no treatment has been established as having clear-cut advantages, considerable controversy exists over a "best approach" to the diagnosis and treatment of breast cancer.

---

*1% of breast carcinomas occur in men

However, one point has been agreed upon. When treatment is initiated, the stage to which the disease has progressed can be correlated with the patient's prognosis. A growing concern has developed for earlier and earlier diagnosis so that survival can be improved. Diagnostic methods are being developed for use in helping plan more rational treatment for breast cancer and for assessing the results of such treatment. Such diagnostic methods also permit breast cancer patients to be followed closely for evidence of recurrent metastatic disease.

A revolution is underway in medicine. A particularly vigorous facet of this revolution is concerned with breast cancer. The call for a more rational approach to breast cancer diagnosis and therapy is being joined by those with the greatest commitment, women (3) who have or may develop the disease.

In this volume, a review is presented of current diagnostic methods with emphasis on the place of nuclear medical imaging as applied to breast carcinoma. A reasonable diagnostic and therapeutic approach to the patient is presented along with an assessment of the expected yield from the wide range of potential tests. Generally, these tests are innocuous and it is tempting to over use them. However, only those with a strong liklihood of contributing to the patient's diagnosis and care should be performed. In the instance of mammography, the relatively high radiation exposure is also a consideration for limiting the application of this useful procedure.

Permission to use these patient studies and x-rays was generously granted by Dr. John L. Doppman, Chief, Department of Radiology, Clinical Center and Dr. Douglass C. Tormey, Medical Oncology Section, Medicine Branch National Cancer Institute.

Dr. Stanley Levenson, Mae F. Go, Dr. Julie E. Timins helped in preparation of the manuscript. All scintigraphs were obtained with the expert technical help of Janice H. Bird, Camille L. Boyce, Elizabeth L. Evans, Eung T. Lee, Eleanor J. Myers and Sybil J. Swann. The manuscript was typed by Phyllis E. Metzger, with the assistance of Luella Bentz, and Paula K. McPherson.

(1) Seidman, H. Cancer of the breast: statistical and epidemiological data. Cancer, 24: 1355, 1969.

(2) Halsted, W.S. The results of radical operations for the cure of cancer of the breast. Ann Surg. 46: 80, 1907.

(3) Kushner, R. Breast cancer. Harcourt, Brace, Jovanovich, New York, 1975.

CONTENTS

CHAPTER 1

Diagnostic Considerations in Breast Cancer

Douglass C. Tormey, M.D., Ph.D.
James N. Ingle, M.D.
Medical Oncology, Medicine Branch
National Cancer Institute
National Institutes of Health
Bethesda, Maryland

The breast is the most common site of female malignancy in the United States, with carcinoma of the breast the leading cause of mortality due to cancer in women between the ages of 15-74 years (1). In the age group, 40-44, breast cancer is responsible for more deaths than all other causes (2). The American Cancer Society estimates that 90,000 women were diagnosed as having breast cancer and 32,000 women died of the disease during 1974.

The most important prognostic factor at the time of presentation is the extent of disease. A reduction in early fatality rates was noted in patients screened periodically with clinical examination and mammography (3). It would be desirable to extend the concepts of earlier diagnosis and appropriate treatment to all breast cancer patients, regardless of their disease stage.

Since there are no universal guidelines for the evaluation and follow-up of patients with suspected, primary, or metastatic disease, this discussion will present our views and those in the literature concerning diagnostic concepts and procedures. Emphasis will be placed on nuclear medicine techniques. Three general clinical settings will be considered: (A) the patient with a suspicious breast lesion, (B) the patient with proven primary breast cancer and, (C) the patient with recurrent or metastatic disease.

A. The Patient with a Breast Lesion

The patient with a breast mass, nipple discharge or some other complaint should be evaluated in a manner dictated by the history and physical examination. For example, in cases of nipple discharge, cytologic examination is indicated. Techniques are being developed to obtain material from the nipple with a breast suction pump and ductal cannulation. Those patients with a breast mass or suspicious skin changes should be evaluated with diagnostic procedures directed at further characterizing the breast lesion (Figure 1). As the sensitivity of the clinical examination is observer dependent, procedures such as mammography, xeroradiography, thermography and ultrasonotomography are utilized to improve diagnostic accuracy. When comparing clinical examination, mammography and thermography in 306 histologically confirmed breast cancers, the detection sensitivity of these modalities was 82%, 85%, and 72%, respectively (4). When clinical examination was combined with mammography, the accuracy increased to 92%. Ultrasonotomography, a relatively new procedure, has been reported capable of diagnosing breast cancer in 90% of cases (5); sensitivity for lesions less than 2 cms. was 82%. Breast scintigraphy, another modality, demonstrates 99mTc pertechnetate (6) and 67Ga localization in malignant breast tumors. Unfortunately, a significant incidence of false-positive and false-negative studies occur. This latter technique is fully discussed in Chapter 4. Of the aforementioned ancillary procedures, the mammogram is used most commonly and is discussed in Chapter 7 (Roentgenographic and Other Procedures).

In those patients with a high clinical suspicion of malignancy, an adequate histologic tissue specimen is necessary. Needle biopsy and needle aspiration are ideal procedures for this in view of their simplicity and low morbidity; neither appears to adversely affect patient survival (7,8). If either of these techniques is positive for malignancy, the patient should be fully evaluated for metastatic disease prior to definitive surgery (Table 1, Column 3). Essentially the same format is required in patients with a negative needle aspirate prior to biopsy under general anesthesia, followed by definitive surgery if the biopsy is positive (Table 1, Column 2). However, if the biopsy is performed several days prior to mastectomy, the extensive diagnostic testing can be postponed until biopsy results return (Table 1, Column 1). Table 1 does not include those studies performed on a routine pre-operative basis for the evaluation of cardiac, renal, metabolic and coagulation status. The importance of this preliminary evaluation is paramount, for the presence of metastatic disease dramatically alters therapy. Local surgical intervention may be modified and some form of systemic therapy instituted at an earlier date.

In these settings, patient evaluation is based upon the location of known metastatic disease. The distribution for disease sites varies among the literature. In one autopsy series, the major sites of metastases were: lung (77%); bone (75%); mediastinal lymph nodes (66%); pleura (65%); liver (61%); adrenals (54%); peritoneal and retroperitoneal lymph nodes (44%); pericardium (35%); brain (29%); peritoneum (25%); diaphragm (25%) and ovaries (23%) (9). For the purpose of planning a diagnostic protocol, however, of utmost

TABLE 1

DIAGNOSTIC PROCEDURES IN PATIENTS WITH SUSPECTED OR PROVEN PRIMARY BREAST CARCINOMA

Procedures	Prebiopsy Diagnosis Unknown	Preoperative Diagnosis Unknown	Preoperative Post Biopsy Diagnosis Cancer
History	x	x	x
Physical Examination	x	x	x
Mammogram or Xeroradiograph	x	x	x
CBC	x	x	x
Alkaline Phosphatase		x	x
SGOT or SGPT, Bilirubin		x	x
Chest X-ray		x	x
Needle Aspiration of Breast	x		
Biopsy of Breast Lesion	x		
Bone Scan		x	x
X-rays of Abnormal Areas on Bone Scan		x	x
Liver Scan		x[1]	x[1]
Brain Scan		x[2]	x[2]

[1]If abnormality of liver on physical examination or function tests
[2]If indicated by clinical abnormality

importance is the anatomic region of first recurrence. A study of 305 post-radical mastectomy patients, with and without three days of post-operative chemotherapy, demonstrated the following statistical distribution of first recurrence sites: integument (31%); skeletal (26%); respiratory (19%); lymphatic (13%); digestive (9%); ovaries (1%); and brain (1%) (10). Data for the groups were comparable, with the exception of a slightly lower incidence of skeletal metastases (21%) in the group not receiving chemotherapy. The necessity for a thorough evaluation of these systems and organs is then quite apparent.

Of critical interest, both prognostically and therapeutically in any patient with a breast lesion, is the skeletal examination. Advocated by many, with some variations, a skeletal survey consisting of a lateral skull view, A-P and lateral radiographs of the thoraco-lumbar spine, as well as A-P pelvic images could be performed. The entire radiographic approach employed at the National Institues of Health is described in Chapter 7. Suffice it to say, the plain X-ray is considered an insensitive procedure for evaluating these major sites of osseous metastases (11).

Bone scintigraphy, in contrast, has been found superior to roentgenographic procedures by numerous investigators. A review of the literature is presented in Chapter 5 (Skeletal Scintigraphy). Controversy, however, still exists concerning the value of routine pre-operative bone scanning and the metastatic survey. Robbins reported in 1972 (12) and reiterated in 1974 (13), that these procedures are indicated only in patients with bone pain, or when a primary lesion greater than 5 cms. in diameter is accompanied by extensive axillary metastases. This contention was based on the analysis of over 300 potentially curable breast cancer patients, of whom only 19% developed osseous metastases within 10 years of their primary surgery. The justification for these techniques would be their utility in the decision for mastectomy.

Contradictory information was obtained by Galasko (14), who evaluated fluorine-18 bone scintigraphy in 50 pre-operative patients with breast carcinoma. In no instance was metastatic disease detectable either clinically or radiologically. Radiographs of the lateral skull, as well as cervical, thoracic, lumbar spine, and P-A pelvis were obtained. Primary tumors ranged in size from less than 2 cms. to larger than 5 cms. in their greatest dimension. All patients had either no palpable ipsilateral axillary nodes or movable ipsilateral axillary lymph nodes. Twelve (24%) were found to have bone scan abnormalities suggestive of metastatic disease. Lesions in 10 of these 12 patients were subsequently visualized roentgenographically or confirmed at autopsy. No correlation was made between primary tumor size, nodal status and bone scan findings.

Current evidence would suggest the use of bone scanning in preference to the roentgenographic survey in a patient with suspected carcinoma of the breast prior to biopsy and definitive surgery. While the yield may be low, potentially significant baseline images are available for future reference. Gerber et al. (15) reported a 5% incidence of positive pre-operative 99mTc diphosphonate bone scans in 109 patients with Stage I or II breast carcinoma. During the 3-24 month post-operative period, follow-up studies in 48 women demonstrated scan conversion from normal to abnormal in 11 (23%). Of this group, 73% were post-menopausal. Both pre-operative baseline and serial post-operative bone scanning were recommended. If a scintigraphic abnormality is discovered, roentgenographic correlation is advisable. In cases of a positive bone scan with negative roentgenograms, tomography will frequently demonstrate disease. The thoroughness of this approach has provided sites for bone biopsy, thus establishing a definitive diagnosis.

In evaluating the liver, routine biochemical tests include alkaline phosphatase, bilirubin, SGOT and SGPT. There is disagreement concerning the indications for liver scanning. It is well accepted that in the patient with a known malignancy, the liver scan can provide visible evidence for metastases. This is most often observed in the presence of abnormal liver function tests and/or hepatomegaly. Still in question is the value of liver scintigraphy in the presence of normal liver function tests and physical examination. Poulose et al. (16), in an evaluation of a variety of primary neoplasms, recommended liver scanning prior to major tumor surgery in every patient, including those with unremarkable physical and biochemical hepatic findings. Excluding the bromsulphalein (BSP) dye test, 33% of 54 patients with hepatic metastases demonstrated as many as four normal biochemical liver function tests. In addition, livers of normal size were noted in 54% of 104 necropsy patients with metastatic liver disease. In contrast, Rosenthal and Kaufman (17) reported nine false-negative scans in 10 patients with documented liver metastases; liver function tests and hepatic examination were normal. In 62 other patients with no evidence for secondary neoplasm, the scan was falsely abnormal or equivocal in seven. Biochemical and clinical parameters were again normal.

While the sensitivity of this procedure relative to biochemical tests and physical examination may prove a valuable baseline procedure, routine liver scintigraphy in patients with suspected breast cancer has not been rewarding. The experience and approach in our protocol setting is described in Chapter 2 (Liver Scintigraphy).

Brain scanning, while a useful tool in the detection and confirmation of cerebral metastases, is indicated only in the

TABLE 2

PERCENT RECURRENCE RATES IN BREAST CANCER PATIENTS ACCORDING TO IPSILATERAL AXILLARY LYMPH NODE STATUS AT TIME OF MASTECTOMY

Nodes		Time After Mastectomy		
Status	Number	18 Months	5 Years	10 Years
Negative	-	5%	21%	24%
Positive	1-3	16%	49%	65%
Positive	>3	44%	81%	86%

presence of neurological signs or symptoms. Although Quinn described the excellent sensitivity of brain scanning in 32 of 34 patients with proven intracerebral breast metastases (18), its value as a routine screening agent in our patient population has not been demonstrated (Chapter 3, Brain Scintigraphy).

Whole body 67Ga scanning has also been studied in breast cancer. Richman et al. (19), retrospectively evaluated the utility of 67Ga scintigraphy in 125 primary and metastatic breast carcinoma patients (Chapter 6). With rare exception, this scintigraphic procedure demonstrated only corroborative capabilities and was inferior to individual organ tracer studies. Gallium-67 scintigraphy is not recommended in the absence of metastatic disease.

B. Proven Primary Breast Cancer

The goal of the post-operative follow-up program is to detect disease recurrence at the earliest possible date. The intensity of this program should be determined by the risk of recurrence. At the present time, ipsilateral axillary nodal status at mastectomy appears to be the most reliable single prognostic indicator. Fisher et al. (20,21) have classified the lymph node status of these patients as follows: (1) negative nodes, (2) 1 to 3 positive nodes, and (3) greater than 3 positive nodes. The recurrence rates of these groups of patients are markedly different (Table 2).

With these considerations, a follow-up program is proposed in Tables 3 and 4. For the first five years following mastectomy, intensive efforts are undertaken to detect recurrent or metastatic disease (Table 3); in the ensuing 5-10 years (Table 4), the follow-up program can usually be relaxed. Although the majority of patients with positive axillary lymph nodes at the time of mastectomy demonstrate recurrence within the first five post-operative years, a significant number will also relapse during the second five year period. Since patients with negative lymph nodes have a low recurrence rate during the 5 to 10 year period, bone scans and chest roentgenograms can probably be eliminated as routine procedures in this group. The determining factor in these situations remains at the physician's discretion. After 10 years patients will continue to relapse, but most can probably be followed with an annual history, physical examination and blood studies as noted in Table 3. In those women with a history of positive axillary nodes, yearly chest roentgenograms and bone scans are suggested. Ideally, all follow-up programs should minimize inconvenience, discomfort and psychological stress to the patient, without sacrificing an early diagnosis of recurrence.

Concerning the asymptomatic patient, roentgenograms should be performed after identification of abnormal areas on bone scan.

TABLE 3

POSTOPERATIVE FOLLOW-UP OF PATIENTS WITH NO EVIDENCE OF RESIDUAL CANCER DURING THE FIRST FIVE YEARS AFTER MASTECTOMY

(Intervals in Months)

	Negative Nodes	Positive Nodes	
		1 to 3	>3
History	6	3 to 6	3
Physical Examination	6	3 to 6	3
CBC	12	6	3
SGOT or SGPT	12	6	3
Alkaline Phosphatase	12	6	3
Chest X-ray	12	6	3
Bone Scan	12	6	3

TABLE 4

FOLLOW-UP PROGRAM FOR PATIENTS WITH NO EVIDENCE OF RESIDUAL CANCER FROM FIVE TO TEN YEARS AFTER MASTECTOMY

(Intervals in Months)

	Negative Nodes	Positive Nodes	
		1 to 3	>3
History	6	6	6
Physical Examination	6	6	6
CBC	12	12	12
SGOT or SGPT	12	12	12
Alkaline Phosphatase	12	12	12
Chest X-ray	-	12	12
Bone Scan	-	12	12

Liver and brain scans do not appear to be effective screening tests for recurrent disease and need only be performed if clinically indicated. Although the patient with a history of cancer in one breast is at higher risk of developing cancer in the other breast than the general population, this occurs at a relatively low rate of 1% per year. Routine mammography should probably be reserved for select high risk patients, such as those with a more aggressive type of primary disease.

Biochemical tumor marker studies are also of interest in patients with proven primary breast cancer. While still in the preliminary stages of evaluation, elevated serum carcinoembryonic antigen (CEA) values were noted in several cases of resected, apparently localized primary carcinoma of the breast (22,23). Although non-specific, these findings may suggest this test as potentially more sensitive than conventional diagnostic modalities.

C. Recurrent or Metastatic Disease

Once the patient has disseminated disease, the frequency of follow-up is increased. This course is chosen to ascertain treatment failures with dispatch. Hopefully, more effective therapy can then be instituted. The frequency of these procedures is directly related to the types of therapy. For example, a complete blood count may be obtained once a month with hormonal therapy, but weekly intervals would be more preferable with some combination chemotherapy regimens. A basic follow-up program is outlined in Table 5.

Regarding imaging procedures for skeletal evaluation, the bone scan provides greater sensitivity in the detection of new lesions, while skeletal roentgenograms are more sensitive for following sites of known disease. Concepts concerning diagnostic imaging procedures in patients with skeletal metastases are elaborated upon in Chapter 5 (Skeletal Scintigraphy).

Other tests have a variable degree of utility in the follow-up evaluation of metastatic breast disease. The liver scan, when abnormal, rarely contributes significantly to patient management unless a lesion of greater than 5 cms. is present (24). Despite these limitations, a baseline liver scan in the patient with known metastatic disease is recommended. This may provide useful information should the patient subsequently develop abnormalities in liver function tests or physical examination. Irregularities by either of these parameters warrants liver scintigraphy. When metastases are demonstrated, progressive disease and response to therapy can be evaluated. Baseline or routine brain scanning without neurological manifestations is not advocated in this clinical setting. It has been our experience that this procedure does not provide significant information. Gallium-67 scanning, as

TABLE 5

FOLLOW-UP INTERVALS IN PATIENTS WITH METASTATIC CARCINOMA OF THE BREAST

Test	Intervals (Weeks)
History	1-4
Physical Examination	1-4
CBC	1-4
SGOT or SGPT	4
Alkaline Phosphatase	4
Chest X-ray	8-12
Bone Scan	12
X-rays of abnormal areas being monitored and new abnormalities on bone scan	12

previously noted, rarely contributes to the data gained by other modalities. However, it has been more sensitive than mediastinal tomography in detecting mediastinal lesions in several cases (19) (Chapter 6). Whole body 67Ga scintigraphy is not presently recommended as a routine test. Mammography also seldom provides objectively measurable parameters. A bone marrow biopsy may be helpful for guiding the use of chemotherapy, although its value in follow-up is unknown. As a diagnostic tool in breast cancer patients, however, it is considerably more sensitive than a bone marrow aspirate (25). A BSP test is potentially useful if other liver function tests are normal, although its importance in follow-up could be lessened by the effects of chemotherapy. The value of tumor markers such as CEA, in the setting of metastatic disease, has not been established; nevertheless, a favorable clinical response was accompanied by a decrease in abnormally elevated CEA levels in several breast cancer patients (22,25).

Of final note is the topic of estrogen receptor analysis, a subject which applies to both primary and metastatic breast carcinoma patients. This field of study has been comprehensively covered in detail by McGuire et al. (26). Whenever tumor tissue is available for biopsy, either prior to or during a therapeutic maneuver, recent evidence suggests the advisability of submitting a portion of the specimen for estrogen receptor analysis. Depending upon the technique utilized, the assay can be performed with as little as 10 mg. of tissue in most situations; however, 200-500 mgs. of tissue are occasionally required. Suffice it to say, an experienced laboratory is necessary.

The presence or absence of estrogen receptor binding protein appears to have prognostic ramifications for the subsequent response of the patient to various types of hormonal manipulation. Among the modes of endocrine intervention are: adrenalectomy, oophorectomy, and hypophysectomy, as well as exogenous therapy with estrogens, androgens, or corticosteroids. If no estrogen receptor is present, the probability of remission induction with these procedures is 5-10%. When the estrogen receptor protein is found, there is a marked increase in the likelihood of response to either surgical or exogenous hormonal therapy; 50-65% of this group have achieved remission under these circumstances. At present, there is no correlation between the estrogen receptor status (quantitatively or qualitatively), the duration of the post-operative disease-free interval, or the durability of any response obtained in metastatic disease. Intensive efforts are continuing in this most interesting field of study.

In summary, there are numerous approaches and modalities for evaluating patients with a suspicious breast lesion, proven primary breast cancer, and recurrent or metastatic disease. The nuclear medicine procedure best serving these patients appears to be whole body skeletal scintigraphy. Liver, brain and 67Ga scintigraphy should be selectively applied to high risk patients and in those situations where clinical or biochemical evidence is suggestive of disease.

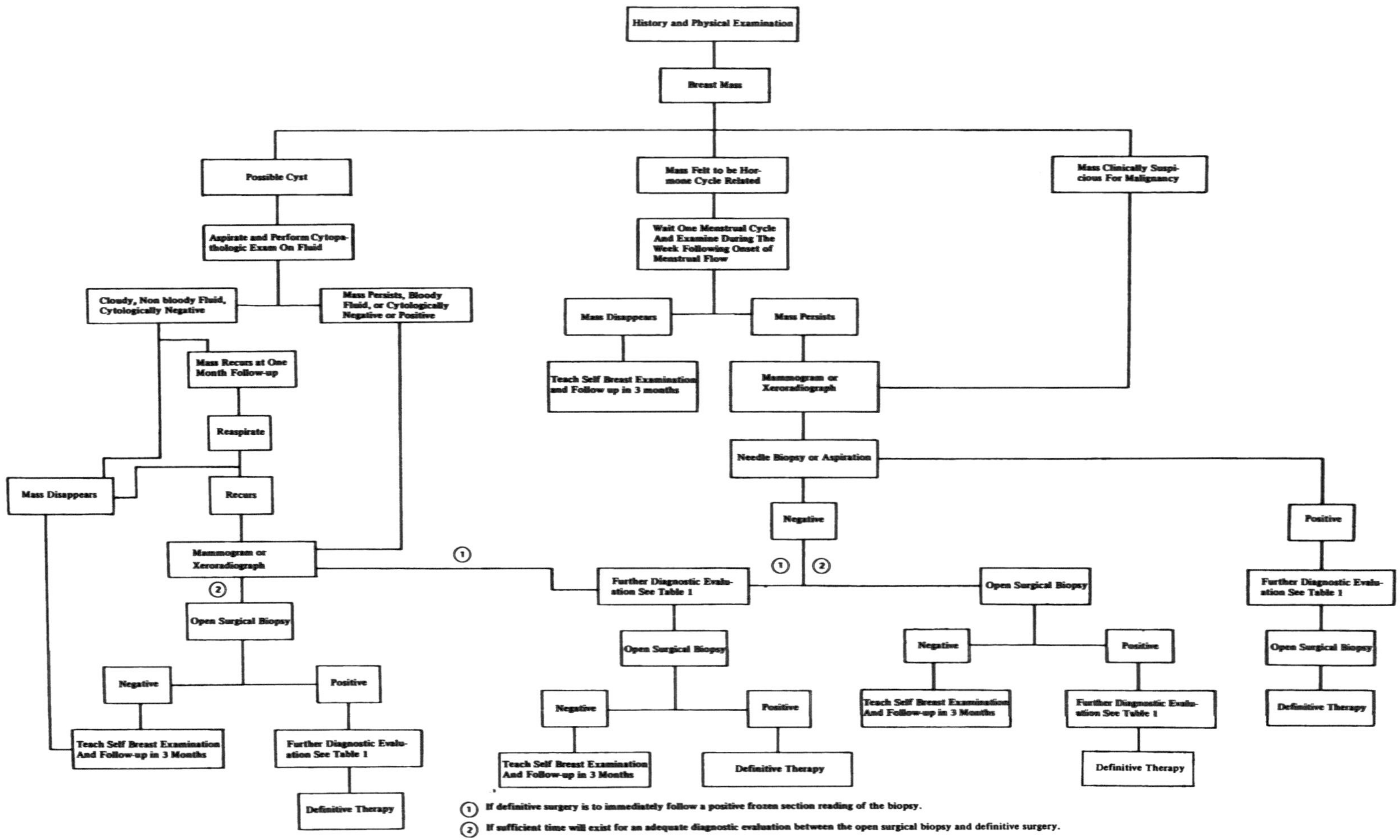

Fig. 1-1. Diagnostic flow in patients with a breast mass.

References Chapter 1

1. U. S. Public Health Service, National Vital Statistics Division: Vital Statistics of the United States, Annual 1930-1968. Washington U. S. Government Printing Office, 1934-71.

2. Silverberg, D., Holleb, A.I. Cancer Statistics - 1971. Cancer 21: 13, 1971.

3. Shapiro, S., Strax, P., Venet, L. Periodic breast cancer screening in reducing mortality from breast cancer. JAMA 215: 1777, 1971.

4. Isard, H., Becker, W., Shilo, R., Ostrum, B. Breast thermography after four years and 10,000 studies. Amer J Roentgenol 115: 811, 1972.

5. Kobayashi, T., Takatani, O., Hattori, N., Kimura, K. Differential diagnosis of breast tumors. The sensitivity graded method of ultrasonotomography and clinical evaluation of its diagnostic accuracy. Cancer 33: 940, 1974.

6. Villarreal, R.L., Parkey, R.W., Bonte, F.J. Experimental pertechnetate mammography. Radiology 111: 657, 1974.

7. Berg, J.W., Robbins, G.F. A late look at the safety of aspiration biopsy. Cancer 15: 826, 1962.

8. Robbins, G.F., Brothers, J.H., Eberhart, W.F., Quan, S. Is aspiration biopsy of breast cancer dangerous to the patient? Cancer 7: 774, 1954.

9. Abrams, H.L., Spiro, R., Goldstein, N. Metastases in carcinoma. Analysis of 1000 autopsied cases. Cancer 3: 74, 1950.

10. Fisher, B., Ravdin, R.G., Ausman, R.K., Slack, N.H., Moore, G.E., Noer, R.J. Surgical adjuvant chemotherapy in cancer of the breast: Results of a decade of cooperative investigation. Ann Surg 168: 337, 1968.

11. Edelstyn, G.A., Gillespie, P.J., Grebbell, F.S. The radiological demonstration of osseous metastases. Experimental observations. Clin Radiol 18: 158, 1967.

12. Robbins, G.F., Knapper, W.H., Barrie, J., Kripalani, I., Lawrence, J. Metastatic bone disease developing in patients with potentially curable breast cancer. Cancer 29: 1702, 1972.

13. Robbins, G.F. The rationale for the treatment of women with potentially curable breast carcinoma. Surg Clin North America 54: 793, 1974.

14. Galasko, C.S.B. Skeletal metastases and mammary cancer. Ann Roy Coll Surg Engl 50: 3, 1972.

15. Gerber, F.H., Goodreau, J.J., Kirchner, P.T. Tc-99m-EHDP bone scanning in breast carcinoma. J Nucl Med 16: 529, 1975.

16. Poulose, K.P., Reba, R.C., Deland, F.H., Wagner, H.N. Role of liver scanning in the preoperative evaluation of patients with cancer. Brit Med J 4: 585, 1969.

17. Rosenthal, S., Kaufman, S. The liver scan in metastatic disease. Arch Surg 106: 656, 1973.

18. Quinn III, J.S. Use of diagnostic nuclear medicine procedures in breast cancer. Cancer 28: 1695, 1971.

19. Richman, S.D., Brodey, P.A., Frankel, R.S., De Moss, E.V., Tormey, D.C. Johnston, G.S. Breast scintigraphy with 99mTc pertechnetate and 67Ga citrate. J Nucl Med 16: 293, 1975.

20. Fisher, B., Slack, N.H., Bross, I.D.J. Cancer of the breast: Size of neoplasm and prognosis. Cancer 24: 1071, 1969.

21. Fisher, B. A report to the profession from the Breast Cancer Task Force of the National Cancer Institute, Bethesda, Maryland, National Institutes of Health, September 30, 1974.

22. Steward, A.M., Nixon, D., Zamcheck, N., Aisenberg, A. Carcinoembryonic antigen in breast cancer patients: Serum levels and disease progress. Cancer 33: 1246, 1974.

23. Tormey, D.C., Waalkes, T.P., Ahmann, D., Gehrke, C.W., Zumwatt, R.W., Snyder, J., Hansen, H. Biologic markers in breast carcinoma. I. Incidence of abnormalities of CEA, HCG, three polyamines, and three minor nucleosides. Cancer 35: 1095, 1975.

24. Moertel, C. Personal communication.

25. Ingle, J., Tormey, D., Bull, J. Bone marrow involvement in breast cancer. Proceedings of the American Association for Cancer Research and of the American Society of Clinical Oncology. 16: 245, 1975.

26. McGuire, W.L., Carbone, P.P., Vollmer, E.P.(eds.) Estrogen receptors in human breast carcinoma. New York, Raven Press, 1975.

CHAPTER 2

Liver Scintigraphy

Stanley Levenson, M.D.

Department of Nuclear Medicine
National Institutes of Health
Bethesda, Maryland

Liver scanning has become an integral part of the diagnosis and management of patients with secondary hepatic neoplasm. Its utility in breast cancer patients is therefore clearly apparent. Metastatic liver disease was present in 51% of cases at autopsy in a series collected by Meissner and Warren (1), ranking the liver along with nodal, lung and skeleton as one of the most frequent sites of secondary neoplasm. Fifteen to twenty percent of patients die as a result of hepatic decompensation with up to 50% having clinically significant involvement (2). Nemoto and Dao found a 38% incidence of liver metastasis in postmenopausal women at adrenalectomy and in 31% of premenopausal patients who underwent therapeutic oophorectomy (3).

Because of the extremely serious nature of this disease, it is crucial to have a noninvasive technique such as liver scanning to evaluate patients at the time of their diagnosis and initial therapy, and to provide an indicator for future follow-up. While visualizing metastatic disease in a clinically suspicious liver is foremost in the mind of the investigator, present-day inherent scanning limitations in the detection of secondary disease require that the lesion be at least 2 cms. in size for visualization (4-8). Special additional problems arise in breast carcinoma patients, because of the increasing popularity of chemotherapy as well as hormonal and local radiotherapy (9).

In addition, with an exclusively female patient population, hepatic related disorders, such as gallbladder disease, may present confusing hepatic defects mistaken for neoplasm (10, 11). An I-131 rose bengal liver scan assists in preventing false-positive diagnoses (12).

It is therefore necessary to judiciously evaluate the liver scan with all available parameters before diagnosing metastatic liver disease. Just as in other patients with a predisposing primary neoplasm, nonhomogeneous tracer distribution without discrete focal filling defects should not be over-interpreted (13). Correlation of suspicious scans with clinical hepatic enlargement or change in hepatic size, as well as incorporation of blood chemistries such as alkaline phosphatase and serum transaminase levels will invariably enhance the diagnostic accuracy of this procedure. Without the scan, abnormal liver function tests are non-specific and can be quite misleading (18). It is well known, however, that metastatic disease, in its own insidious fashion, may be unexpectedly detected in the absence of physical or biochemical manifestations (18,19) (Fig. 2-1). This should encourage heightened awareness on the part of the clinician in young, premenopausal patients, and in those women with a more highly malignant carcinoma, e.g., anaplastic carcinoma. When studies appear equivocal, as they do in many cases, the scintiscan may then be useful as a geographic parameter for liver biopsy (5,12,18). If normal tissue is obtained, as occurs in many patients with questionable, or limited but definite focal disease, peritoneoscopy, using the liver scan as a guide, has been rewarding (20). While hepatic angiography may also be employed following a questionable scan (21,22), it is rarely used for diagnosis in this patient population.

The liver scintigraphic technique that is routinely employed is as follows: patients receive 2 mCi 99mTc sulfur colloid intravenously. Scintiphotos are obtained approximately 10 minutes post-injection in the anterior supine position with right and left costal margin markers. The gamma camera, because of its flexibility and large field of view, has been the instrument of choice for this procedure. The remainder of the images are obtained in the upright position, including a second anterior view which frequently clarifies suspicious regions and provides information regarding liver pliability (23). Right lateral and posterior views are similarly performed, as well as corresponding images of the spleen. Oblique views are obtained in questionable situations. In evaluating the utility of liver scanning in our patient population, scans were performed on a quarterly basis, and more frequently when warranted by the clinical course. Over 600 liver scans were obtained during the two year interval, January 1973 - January 1975.

The abnormalities detected in liver scintiscanning are numerous. One must always be aware of artefacts (10,24,25), and in particular, those in the superior dome on the right lobe secondary to an overlying breast, a breast prosthesis (26), or a portal of radiation (5). This latter finding may also involve both right and left hepatic lobes after extensive irradiation to the thoracic spine. Rib margin indentations can also produce linear hepatic defects which usually assume the contour of the costal margin (5). All the above have been noted to cause generalized decreases in hepatic tracer in the aforementioned regions (Fig. 2-2).

Another not uncommon finding is flattening of the superior dome of the right hepatic lobe (Fig. 2-3). This is frequently, but not always, accompanied by an excessive extension of the liver beneath the right costal margin with palpatory findings indicating hepatomegaly. The presentation of a flattened dome and inferiorly displaced liver should always alert one to the possibility of a pleural effusion or chronic obstructive pulmonary disease as the etiology (27).

Undiagnosed or underlying liver disease can be extremely perplexing in scan interpretation, frequently causing varying degrees of tracer nonhomogeneity and hepatomegaly (5,28)(Fig. 2-4). Again, the imposing influence of a breast carcinoma diagnosis, particularly with bone and/or lymph node metastases, may incorrectly bias the scan interpretation. Hepatic abnormalities secondary to anesthesia induced toxic hepatitis incurred at the time of the patient's mastectomy, hepatic changes associated with systemic chemotherapeutic agents, and serum hepatitis resulting from blood transfusion, demonstrate acute and occasionally chronic changes in the scintiscan. Instances of hepatic fatty infiltration, focal fibrosis and inflammation (etiology unknown) and cirrhosis yield scan images, which in this milieu, would raise the probability of liver metastases. Strict criteria for focal defect interpretation and follow-up scans are suggested.

Liver scanning is also a useful adjunct in elucidating the progression of documented metastases (Figs. 2-5,6,7), and evaluating the response to chemotherapy (Fig. 2-8). While the former is appreciated quite frequently, resolution or significant improvement is also being seen more commonly. Hepatic scintigraphy is now a routine procedure in determining hepatic response to chemotherapy.

As with any form of metastatic liver disease, it is obligatory to evaluate both hepatic lobes. Although the right lobe is more frequently and extensively involved, most probably because of its size and vascularity, the diagnosis of occult disease in the left lobe can radically alter patient therapy (Fig. 2-9).

In certain instances, 67Ga citrate scanning has localized in "cold" areas visualized on the 99mTc sulfur colloid images.

Generally this has not proven to be the case; however, the finding appears to predominate with extensive disease. In the liver, as in other regions of the body, 67Ga has been suboptimal in selectively localizing lesions of metastatic breast carcinoma (Fig. 2-10).

Concerning the spleen, no correlation has been observed with the reported 12% incidence of splenic metastases at autopsy. While images of the spleen are routinely included with liver scintiscans, infiltrative splenic disease has not been visualized. Relative increases in splenic tracer concentration have been seen in patients with significant liver metastases, but, this is the expected finding in cases of severe hepatic compromise due to secondary neoplasm. Four cases of splenomegaly have been observed in our patient population; the etiology is unexplained, since in no instance was hepatic disease evident.

Regarding the sensitivity of liver scanning in patients with known metastatic breast carcinoma, a review of 27 histologically proven cases demonstrated the liver scan as the first index of disease in seven (26%) (30). Abnormal liver function studies and/or physical examination raised the clinician's suspicion in the remaining cases. In no instance was the scan normal in this study group. Other investigators have reported a detection accuracy of 77% in secondary hepatic breast carcinoma; this has been attributed to the interval progression or occurrence of disease between scanning and histopathological documentation, and to the in vivo detection limitations of present-day instrumentation (8).

In conclusion, 99mTc sulfur colloid liver scanning has been found to be an excellent tool in the evaluation of metastatic disease in breast carcinoma patients. It is recommended for the visual documentation of suspected disease, response to chemotherapy, assessing neoplastic progression, and in the presence of abnormal liver function tests, physical evidence for hepatomegaly, or both. Scintigraphic evidence of occult preoperative metastases at the time of presentation should also radically alter surgical plans. This information would then allow a planned approach to the treatment of liver secondaries. On a routine basis, liver scan abnormalities preceded biochemical and physical findings in a significant number of patients. The importance of earlier recognition of metastases and its effect on long-term survival in this age of combination chemotherapy has yet to be determined (31).

Fig. 2-1. At age 32, this patient underwent a right radical mastectomy for infiltrating adenocarcinoma for the breast. There were no positive axillary lymph nodes. A biopsy of the left breast also revealed malignant tissue. Serial studies beginning in July, 1973, demonstrate what appeared to be metastatic changes on February 15, 1974. Percutaneous and peritoneoscopic biopsies were not helpful.

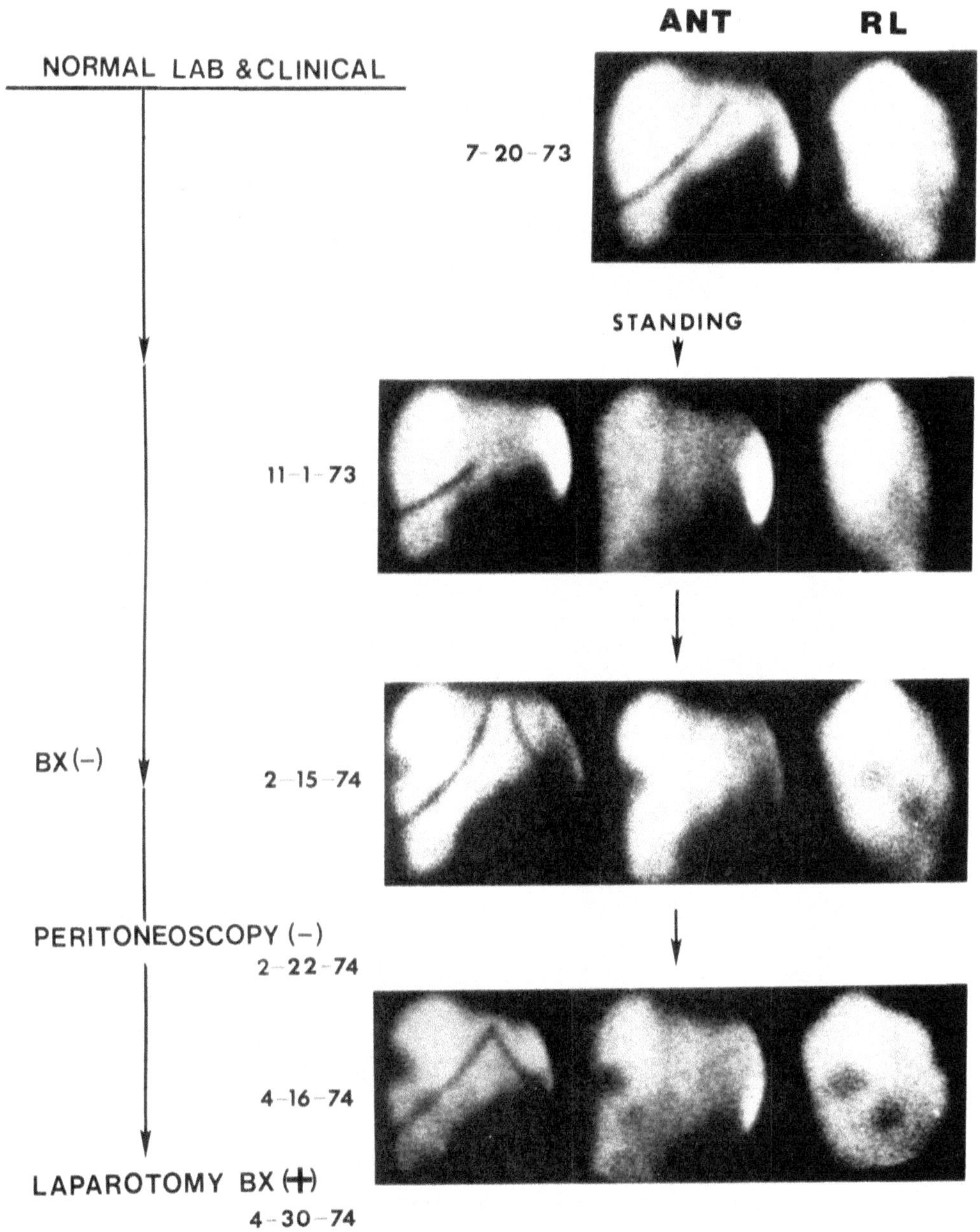

It was not until April 30, 1974, that a biopsy at laparotomy confirmed scan findings. This case exemplifies the detection of metastatic disease by liver scan in the presence of normal liver function tests, physical examination and multiple biopsy attempts. (Ant = anterior reclining, standing = anterior upright, RL = right lateral.)

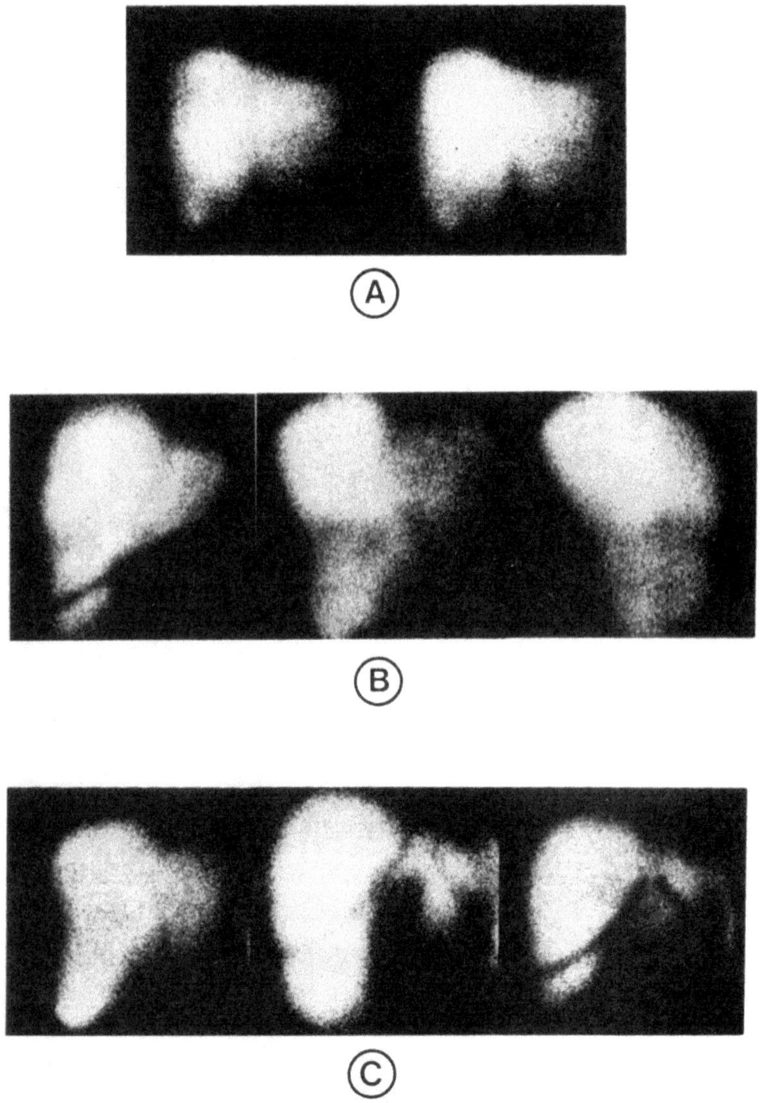

Fig. 2-2. A) An overlying breast or breast prosthesis (left) may decrease the tracer concentration in the superior portion of the right hepatic lobe. This is in contrast to the image in which the artifact has been removed (right). B) Costal compression frequently produces the linear defect seen here in the anterior supine, anterior upright and right lateral projection. C) The pre-vertebral irradiation image (left) is followed by the scan demonstrating a midline tracer decrease following irradiation (middle) and a resolving pattern over the next several months (right). Costal markers are in place on the first scan in (B) and the 2nd and 3rd scans in (C).

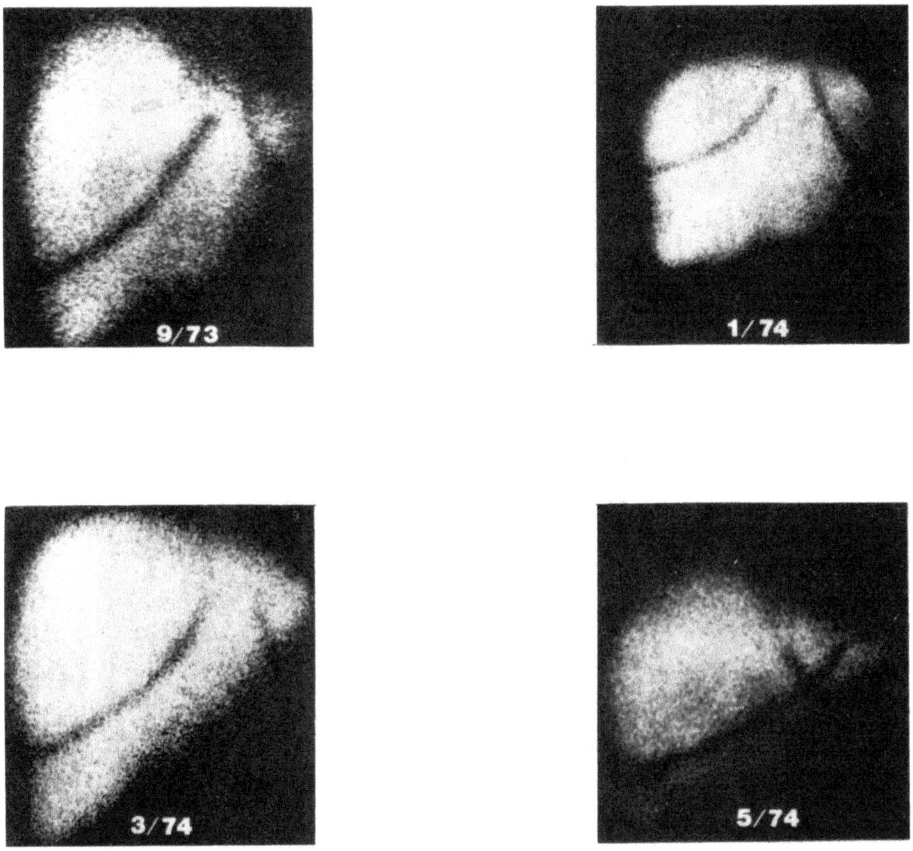

Fig. 2-3. A liver that was somewhat enlarged with nonhomogeneous tracer distribution by scan was followed serially for one year. Bone and bone marrow metastases were first documented in April, 1973, approximately four years after the patient's left radical mastectomy for carcinoma. Pleural effusion with negative cytology in June, 1973, demonstrated malignant cells in January, 1974. Note that the superior dome of the liver progresses from a flattened contour to its normal position and arch with resolution of the pleural fluid following thoracentesis and chemotherapy. Diaphragmatic flattening is also observed in patients with chronic obstructive pulomary disease.

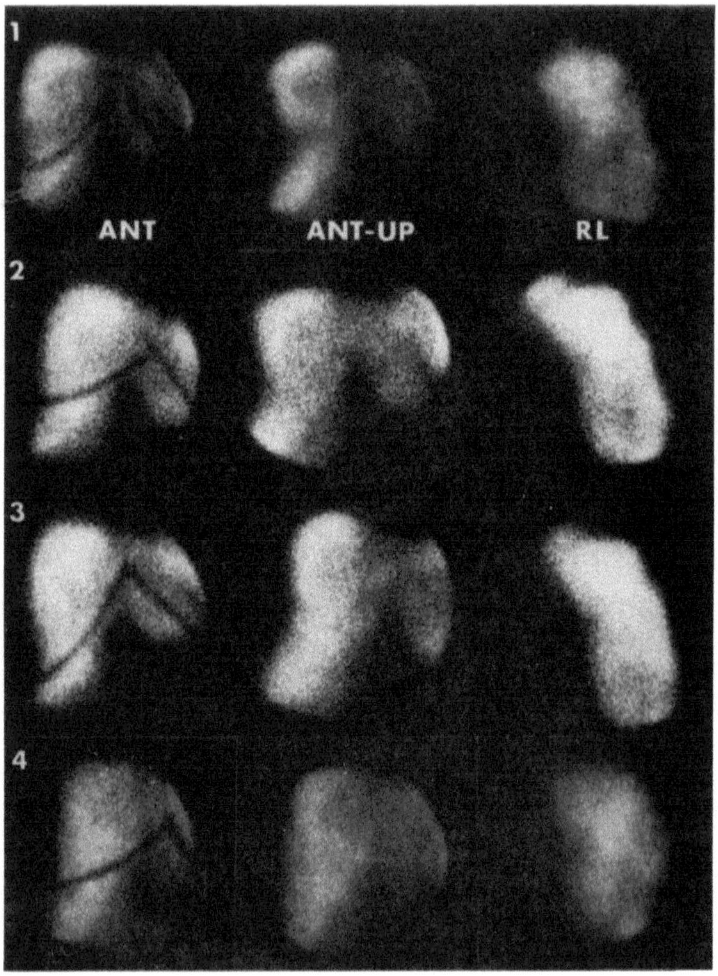

Fig. 2-4. Serial scintiphotos in a patient following her second mastectomy for breast carcinoma demonstrate the potential for scan over-interpretation in this population. The initial study (1) performed five months after mastectomy demonstrated hepatomegaly with nonhomogeneous tracer distribution. The repeat study three months later revealed minimal changes (2). The liver span was 17 cms. in the mid-clavicular line with serum transaminase levels 5-25 times normal. Eight months following the initial study, persistence of the scan findings was noted (3), although enzymes were now normal and the patient was well. Biopsy revealed acute hepatitis, which in retrospect, was thought secondary to halothane toxicity at the time of mastectomy. The final scan (4) obtained one year after the original studies most likely reflects residual hepatic changes. (Ant = anterior supine, Ant-up = anterior upright, RL = right lateral.)

A

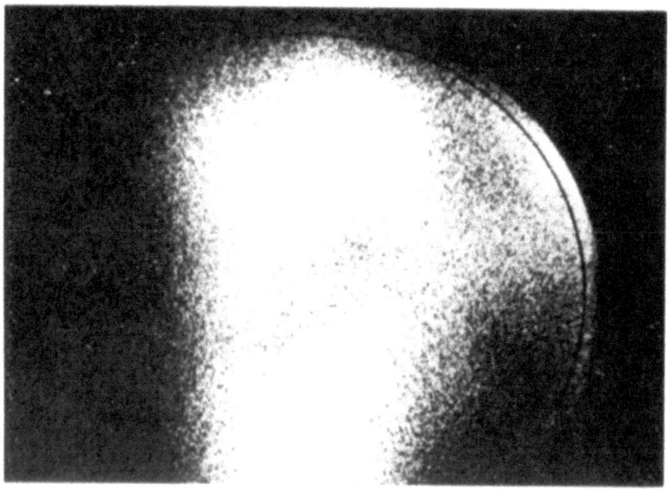

B

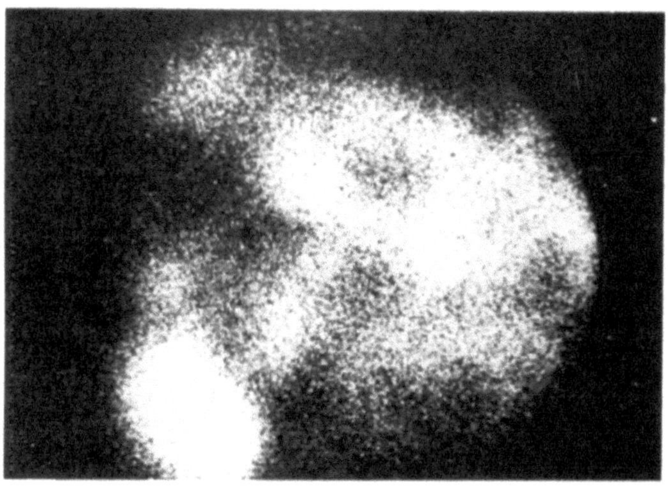

Fig. 2-5. Metastatic liver disease, first documented by scan three years post-radical mastectomy in November 1967, has been followed for almost five years. From 1970 (5A) through 1974 (5B), changes in hepatic scintiphotos have corresponded with the patient's liver function tests, physical findings and general well-being. This most unusual case provides exceptionally long-term followup and survival with severe secondary hepatic involvement.

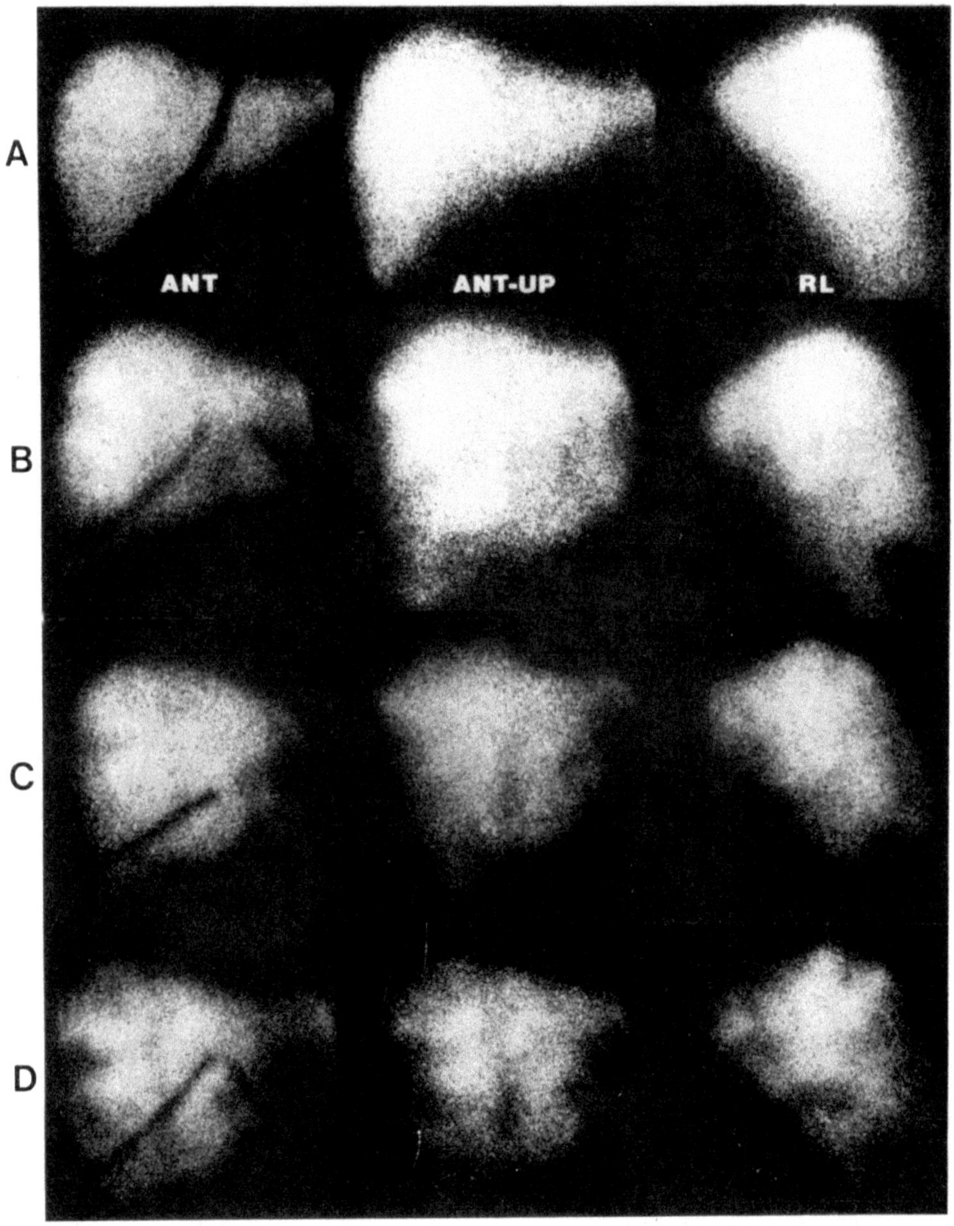

Fig. 2-6. Four liver scans over a one year interval demonstrate the spectrum of appearance of secondary hepatic neoplasm. Normal (6A), nonhomogeneous (6B), patchy (6C), and multiple focal defects (6-D), describe the progressive temporal changes depicted above. Clinical and biochemical parameters were of no assistance. (Ant = anterior reclining, Ant-up = anterior upright, RL= right lateral).

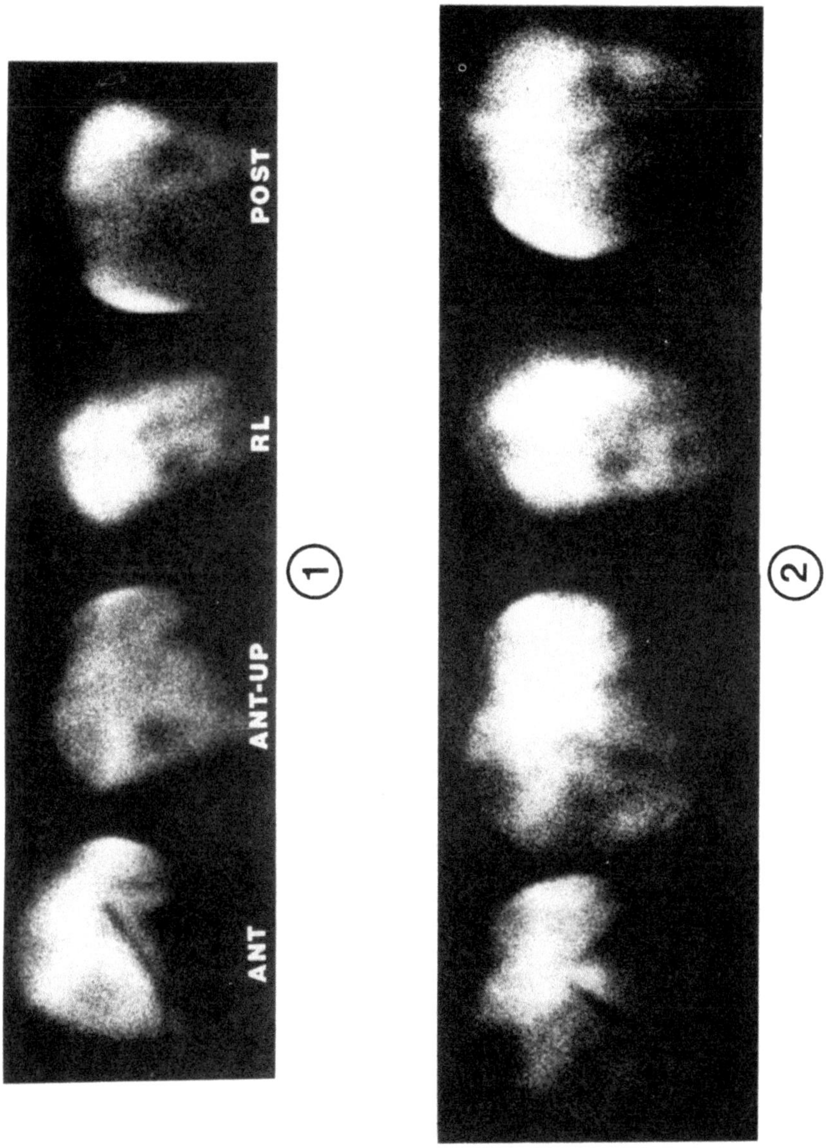

Fig. 2-7. Studies performed seven weeks apart (#1 and #2) demonstrate unusually agressive metastatic disease in a 29 year old post-mastectomy patient.

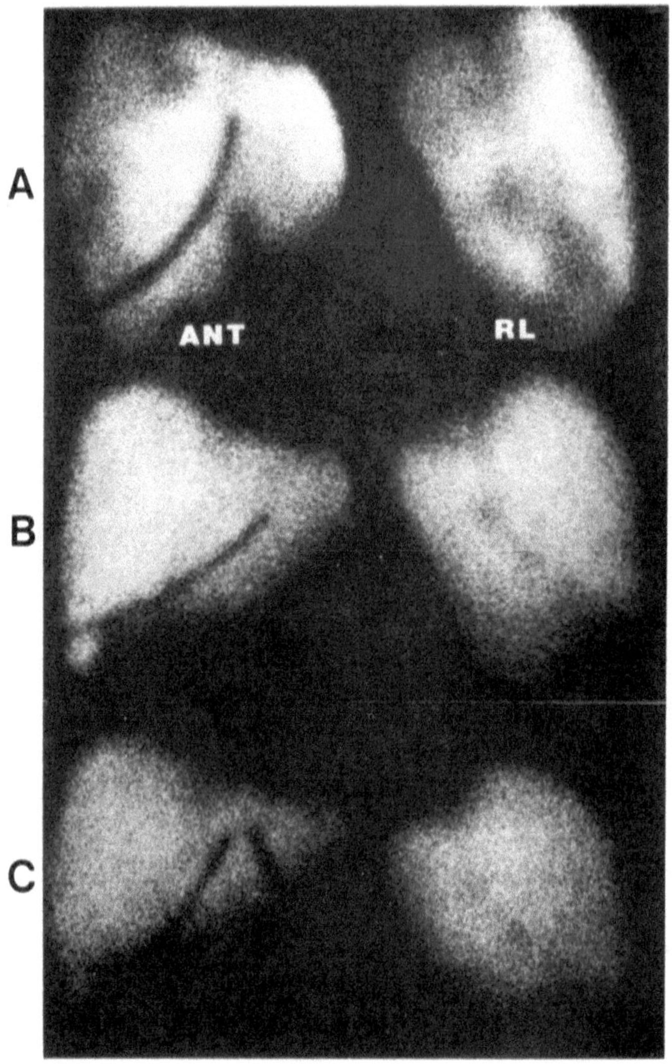

Fig. 2-8. The liver of this patient who has infiltrating ductal cell carcinoma, demonstrates a remarkable response to chemotherapy. Anterior and right lateral images performed initially (A), four (B) and five (C) months following the initiation of therapy demonstrate a dramatic temporal response to chemotherapy. The scan performed after clinical evaluation (A) revealed an enlarging liver with multiple focal filling defects almost certainly representing secondary hepatic neoplasm, although liver function studies were normal. Sequential scans over the five month interval provided the clinician with excellent documentation of the response to therapy in the presence of minimal physical findings and consistently normal liver function text. (Ant = anterior reclining, RL = right lateral.)

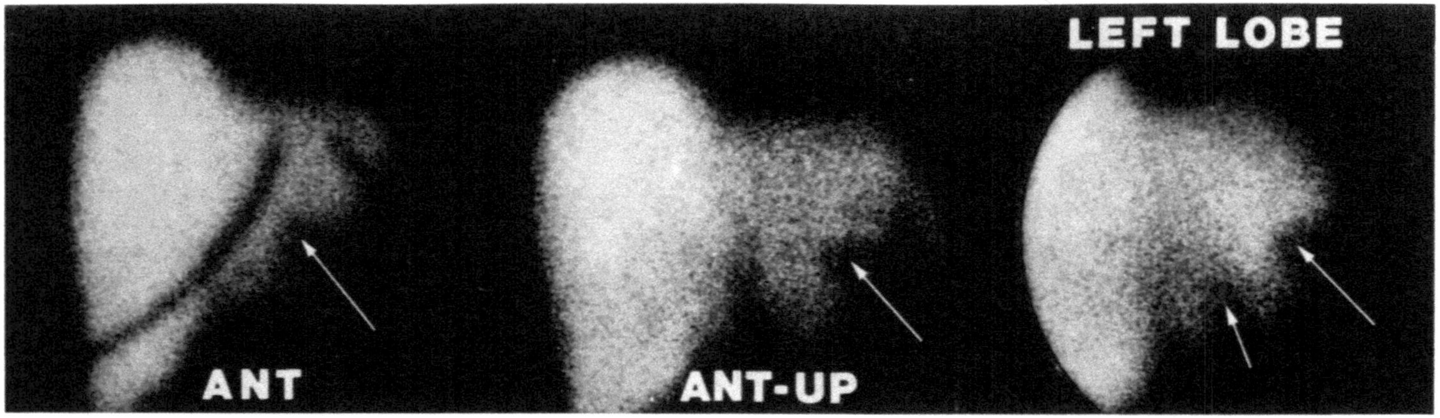

Fig. 2-9. Routine liver scanning in this patient revealed metastatic disease in the left lobe which was easily accessible to periotoneoscopic biopsy. The middle image was performed with the patient in the upright position (ant = anterior reclining, ant-up = anterior upright, left lobe = anterior view of left lobe.)

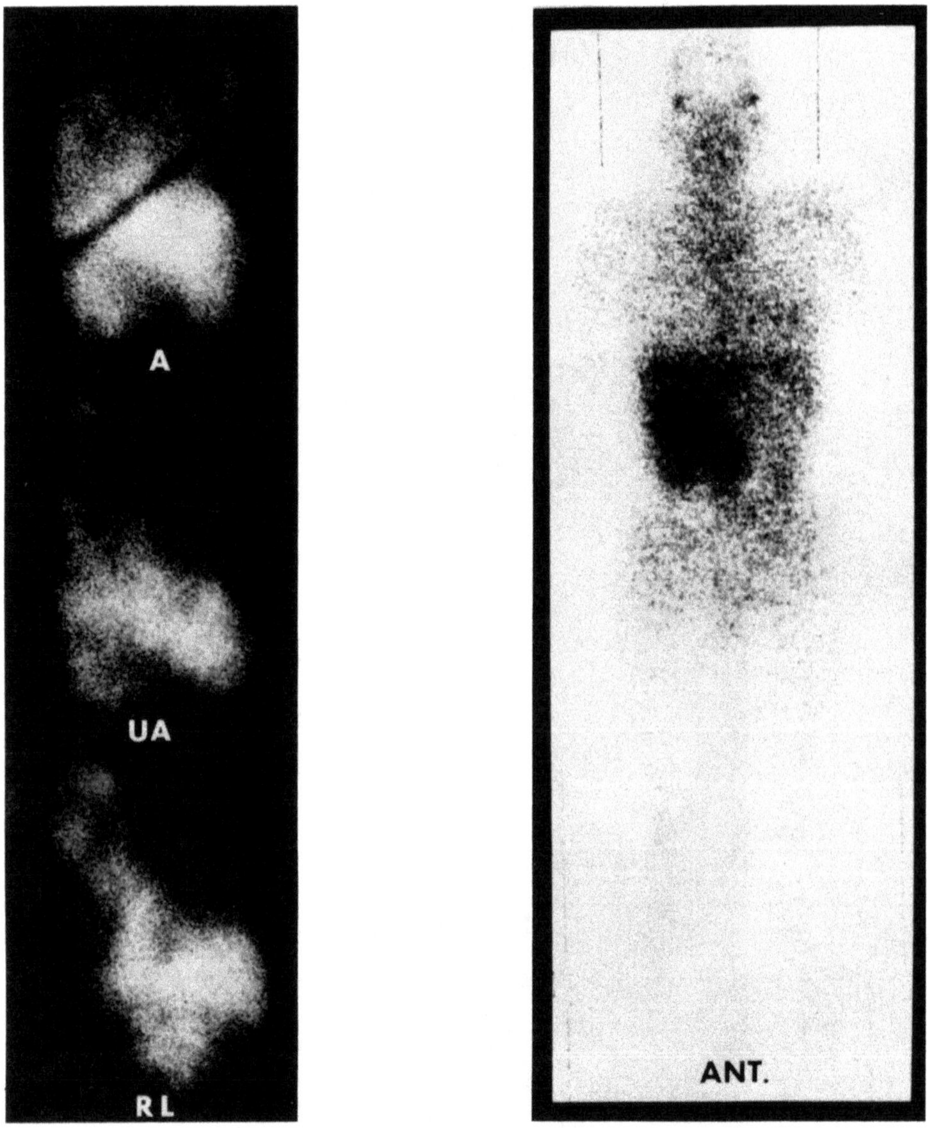

Fig. 2-10. Gallium-67 liver images have not been helpful in patients with carcinoma of the breast. The 99mTc sulfur colloid scan in this patient, revealed metastatic liver disease. Gallium-67 demonstrated no preferential affinity for the sites of metastases and is not recommended in this organ evaluation. (A = anterior reclining, UA = upright anterior, RL = right lateral, ANT = anterior whole body 67Ga rectilinear scan.)

References Chapter 2

1. Meissner, W.A., Warren, S. Sites of metastases at autopsy. In Pathology. Edited by W.A.D. Anderson, St. Louis, C.V. Mosby Co., 1: 538, 1971.

2. Brennan, M.J. Breast cancer. In Cancer Medicine. Edited by J.F. Holland and E. Frei. Philadephia, Lea and Febiger, p. 1785, 1973.

3. Nemoto, T., Dao, T.L. Significance of liver metastasis in women with disseminated breast cancer and undergoing endocrine ablative surgery. Cancer 19: 421, 1966.

4. Wagner, H.N., Jr., McAfee, J.G., Mozley, J.M. Diagnosis of liver disease by radioisotope scanning. Arch Intern Med 107: 324, 1961.

5. McAfee, J., Ause, R.G., Wagner, H.N. Diagnostic value of scintillation scanning of the liver. Arch Intern Med 116: 95, 1965.

6. Johnson, P.M. The Liver. In Clinical Scintillation Scanning. Freeman, L.M. and Johnson, P.M., eds. New York, Harper and Row, p. 260, 1969.

7. Mangum, J.F., Powell, M.R. Liver scintigraphy as an index of liver abnormality. J Nucl Med 14: 484, 1973.

8. Lunia, S., Parthasarathy, K.L., Bakshi, S., Bender, M.A. An evaluation of 99mTc-colloid liver scintiscans and their usefulness in metastatic workup: A review of 1,424 studies. J Nucl Med 16: 62, 1975.

9. Johnston, G.S., Jones, A.E. Sequential liver scanning. J Surg Oncol 1: 205, 1969.

10. Covington, E.E. Pitfalls in liver photoscans. Am J Roentgenol Radium Ther Nucl Med 109: 745, 1970.

11. Covington, E.E. The accuracy of liver photoscans. Am J Roentgenol Radium Ther Nucl Med 109: 742, 1970.

12. Conn, H.O., Spencer, R.P. Observer error in liver scan. Gastroenterology 62: 1085, 1972.

13. Poulose, K.P., Reba, R.C., Cameron, J.L., Wagner, H.N., Jr. The value and limitations of liver scanning for the detection of hepatic metastases in patients with cancer. J Indian Med Assoc 61: 199, 1973.

14. Jhingran, S.G., Jordan, L., Jahns, M.F., Haynie, T.P. Liver scintigrams compared with alkaline phosphatase and BSP determinations in the detection of metastatic carcinoma. J Nucl Med 12: 227, 1971.

15. Gollin, F.F., Sims, J. LeR., Cameron, J.R. Liver scanning and liver function tests. A comparative study. JAMA 187: 111, 1964.

16. Castagna, J., Benfield, J.R., Yamada, H., Johnson, D.E. The reliability of liver scans and function tests in detecting metastases. Surg Gynecol Obstet 134: 463, 1972.

17. Liewendahl, K., Schauman, K.O. Statistical evaluation of liver scanning in combination with liver function tests. Acta Med Scand 192: 395, 1972.

18. Poulose, K.P., Reba, R.C., DeLand, F.H., Wagner, H.N. Role of liver scanning in the preoperative evaluation of patients with cancer. Brit Med J 4: 585, 1969.

19. Davies, R.J., Vernon, M., Croft, D.N. Liver snaps and the detection of clinically unsuspected liver metastases. Lancet 1: 279, 1974.

20. Hitzelberger, A.L., Parker, G.W., Durden, W.D., Johnston, G.S. Peritoneoscopy and radioisotope scintiscanning of the liver in the detection of hepatic metastases. Gastrointestinal Endoscopy, 13: 12, 1967.

21. Jones, A.E., Montgomery, J.L. Utility of combined hepatic scintigraphy and arteriography: Case examples of cirrhosis, hepastoma, and amebic abscess. J Surg Oncol 3: 657, 1971.

22. Freeman, L.M., Bernstein, R.G., Katz, M.C., Derman, A., Meng, C. Combined diagnostic approach of hepatic scanning and celiac angiography in the investigation of liver disease. J Nucl Med 10: 628, 1969.

23. Swann, S.J., Boyce, C.L., Johnston, G.S., Jones, A.E., Hardin, V. Patient positioning for hepatic scintigraphy. J Nucl Med Tech 1: 27, 1973.

24. Volpe, J.A., Morita, E.T., Johnston, G.S. The false positive technetium-99m hepatic scintiscan. J Surg Oncol 1: 345, 1969.

25. Polcyn, R.E., Quinn, J.L., Gottschalk, A. Liver scan artifacts. J Nucl Med 9: 342, 1968.

26. Milder, M.S., Larson, S.M., Swann, S.J. Johnston, G.S. False-positive liver scan due to breast prosthesis. J Nucl Med 14: 198, 1973.

27. Bonte, F.J., Krohmer, J.S., Elmendorf, E., Presley, N.L., Andrews, G.J., Scintillation scanning of the liver: II. Clinical applications. Amer J Roentgenol Radium Ther Nucl Med 88: 275, 1962.

28. Johnson, P.M. Sweeney, W.A. False-positive hepatic scans J Nucl Med 8: 451, 1967.

29. Richman, S.D., Ingle, J.N., Levenson, S.M., Tormey, D.C., Jones, A.E., Johnston, G.S. The usefulness of gallium scintigraphy in primary and metastatic breast carcinoma. J Nucl Med 16: 560, 1975.

30. Levenson, S.M., Ingle, J.N., Richman, S.D., Frankel, R.S., Tormey, D.C., Jones, A.E., Johnston, G.S. Liver scanning in metastatic carcinoma of the breast. J Nucl Med 16: 545, 1975.

31. Mansfield, C.M., Kramer, S., Southard, M.E. The influence of treatment on the survival of patients with hepatic metastases diagnosed by liver scanning. Amer J Roentgenol Radium Ther Nucl Med 109: 749, 1970.

CHAPTER 3

Brain Scintigraphy

Alfred E. Jones, M.D.

Department of Nuclear Medicine
Clinical Center
National Institutes of Health
Bethesda, Maryland

Brain scintigraphy with 99mTc pertechnetate has been used for evaluating patients with breast cancer at the time of the first visit and for follow-up visits. This has proved to be of little value in screening all patients with carcinoma of the breast for possible brain metastases. Brain scanning is more properly applied to the breast carcinoma patient who has neurologic signs or symptoms (Chapter 1: Diagnostic Considerations in Breast Cancer).

The autopsy incidence of breast carcinoma metastatic to brain varies from 10% (1) to 25% (2) and higher (3), while the autopsy incidence of metastatic breast carcinoma involving the skeleton has been reported as being 75% (12). The high incidence of skeletal metastases is reflected by the frequent involvement of the calvarium which in turn, can result in an abnormal 99mTc pertechnetate brain scan (4,5). Thus it is important to determine whether the brain scan abnormality is due to breast carcinoma metastatic to the skull or to the brain or to both sites. This chapter attempts to provide an integrated approach to the use of diphosphonate cranial images, pertechnetate brain scans and 67Ga head views in the detection and differentiation of cerebral breast carcinoma lesions from skull metastases.

In 1967 a scintigraphic approach to separating metastatic lesions of the brain from those of the skull was evaluated using 99mTc pertechnetate and the bone seeking material, ionic strontium-87m. It was observed that 99mTc pertechnetate delineated brain tumors and strontium-87m revealed bone tumors; thus it was suggested that combined studies utilizing both radionuclides in the same subject would be helpful in distinguishing brain tumors from skull tumors (6). This same problem was more recently studied with the newer bone seeking agent 99mTc diphosphonate, which was observed to have a less specific localization within either primary or metastatic neoplasms of the brain than did 99mTc pertechnetate (7).

Nevertheless 99mTc diphosphonate was found to localize in brain lesions and to complicate the interpretation of bone scans of the skull (8). It is known to accumulate in a variety of intracerebral lesions such as cerebral infarction, chronic subdural hematoma, arteriovenous malformation, inflammatory lesions and primary or metastatic neoplasms. Thus while 99mTc pertechnetate has a better tumor-to-brain ratio than 99mTc diphosphonate, the latter agent is far superior in demonstrating metastases to the bony calvarium. Considered in combination, the two scanning agents offer a potential for differentiating breast carcinoma metastatic to the skull from those metastases that are purely intracerebral.

A third agent with greater tumor specificity, such as 67Ga, might prove helpful in cases where 99mTc pertechnetate and 99mTc diphosphonate have provided inconclusive results (9).

As an aid to staging and planning of therapy, patients with breast carcinoma were studied first with a liver scan, then a brain scan, followed by a 99mTc diphosphonate rectilinear bone scan, and finally a whole body rectilinear 67Ga scan. This routine proved especially helpful in evaluating the calvarium and its contents for metastatic breast carcinoma.

Immediately following the liver scan, the patient received 15mCi of 99mTc pertechnetate along with 300 mg. of potassium perchlorate. Thirty to 60 minutes later, a five view gamma camera brain study was performed, collecting 300,000 counts per view.

Whole body bone scans were obtained two days after the 99mTc pertechnetate brain scan, thereby providing enough time for a reasonable clearance of the activity remaining from the brain study. Since the rectilinear bone study provided only anterior and posterior views of the head, additional lateral gamma camera views of the skull and cervical spine were routinely obtained, collecting 50,000 counts per view. Immediately after completion of the bone scan, 67Ga (50uCi/Kg body weight) was administered intravenously and the patient returned 72 hours later for a whole body dual probe rectilinear scan. Gallium-67 head views were not obtained unless there was a suspicious area noted on the brain scan. Since it was recognized that 67Ga was not particularly successful in detecting metastatic breast carcinoma, whole body 67Ga scans were not required of all patients during subsequent scintigraphic follow-up studies (Chapter 1).

Of the N.I.H. patients who came to autopsy, 10 had proven brain metastases. Three of these patients had lesions that were detected by 99mTc pertechnetate brain scintigraphy. One of the three patients had an abnormal 99mTc diphosphonate skull study. In addition, two other patients had positive 99mTc diphosphonate skull views only. Thus five of the 10 patients had abnormal views of the brain or calvarium. Of the remaining five patients one had a lesion in the posterior fossa, a difficult location to detect a lesion by brain scan. The remaining four patients had normal brain and calvarium scans within four weeks of autopsy. At autopsy two of these patients had large lesions and there is no apparent reason why they were not visible on brain scan. Two other patients had lesions that were too small to be seen on brain scan.

The results of the 99mTc pertechnetate brain studies might have been better if views were obtained later than 30 to 60 minutes after dosing (10). This is evident in Fig. 3-1 where 99mTc pertechnetate views at 30 minutes and 90 minutes are compared with 99mTc diphosphonate and 67Ga views of a metastatic breast carcinoma lesion within the brain. Skull views with 99mTc diphosphonate appear to be best four hours after dosing (Fig. 3-2).

Routine 99mTc pertechnetate brain images may show no abnormality in the presence of bony involvement of the calvarium. They should be compared to the rectilinear 99mTc diphosphonate and 67Ga studies and if possible with selected 99mTc diphosphonate gamma camera views of the calvarium (Fig. 3-3). Routine lateral gamma camera views, taken along with the 99mTc diphosphonate whole body rectilinear study, are most productive in revealing and defining the extent of metastatic breast carcinoma within the skull (Chapter 5, Figs. 5-6A and B).

The correlation of brain scan abnormalities with metastases within the calvarium is readily accomplished by comparing the brain scan views with the 99mTc diphosphonate skull views and the skull x-rays (Fig. 3-4). Progression of an abnormal 99mTc pertechnetate study should also be compared with similar 99mTc diphosphonate views and the skull films in order to more reliably credit the change in brain scan to metastatic disease of the skull. Conversely, successful therapy may be demonstrated by serial views of the skull taken before and after therapy (Chapter 5, Fig. 5-5C).

When the bone scans and brain scans are positive in the same area it is possible that contiguous meningeal spread may have occurred since the close application of the dura to the calvarium facilitates direct extension of the malignancy (11). In this group of 10 patients with autopsy proven brain metastasis, two had positive 99mTc diphosphonate skull views and meningeal metastases. One of these two patients also had a left hemiparesis associated with an abnormality on the right seen in the 99mTc pertechnetate brain scan. The diphosphonate image indicated diffuse disease throughout the calvarium in contrast to the 67Ga view which showed a localization within the abnormality detected in the pertechnetate brain scan (Fig. 3-6). The 67Ga appeared to detect the cerebral metastasis and differentiate the brain lesion from the diffuse metastases within the calvarium. Nevertheless, the localization of 67Ga may be no better than that of 99mTc diphosphonate or 99mTc pertechnetate within an intracerebral breast carcinoma metastasis (Fig. 3-1). The variable affinity of 67 Ga for intracerebral breast metastases appears to make it a worthwhile procedure to be employed when the 99mTc pertechnetate study is negative and there is a high suspicion of an intracerebral lesion. A negative 67Ga study offers no reassurance that an intracerebral lesion is not present.

In conclusion, routine 99mTc pertechnetate brain scintigraphy was not a satisfactory screening procedure in the detection of occult cerebral breast carcinoma metastases. Additional gamma camera head views were necessary for a thorough metastatic survey at the time of performing whole body 99mTc diphosphonate bone scans. When the 99mTc pertechnetate brain scan is negative or suspicious in a breast carcinoma patient with neurologic signs or symptoms, gamma camera head views with 99mTc diphosphonate and 67Ga may prove helpful.

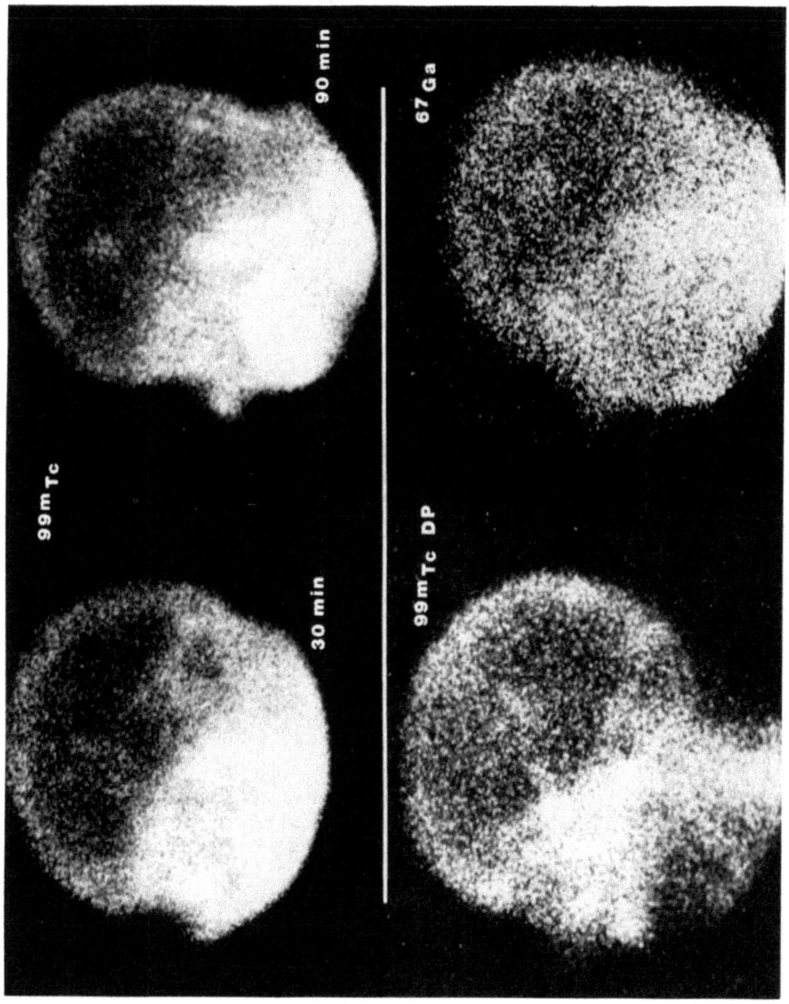

Fig. 3-1. Top: Left lateral images at 30 and 90 minutes following intravenous ^{99m}Tc pertechnetate. Note that this breast carcinoma lesion is seen more clearly at 90 minutes. Bottom: Left lateral ^{99m}Tc diphosphonate and ^{67}Ga images of the same lesion as shown above. Both diphosphonate and ^{67}Ga localized faintly in this lesion. This metastasis demonstrated a poor affinity for ^{67}Ga in contrast to the lesion shown in Figs. 3-7 and 8.

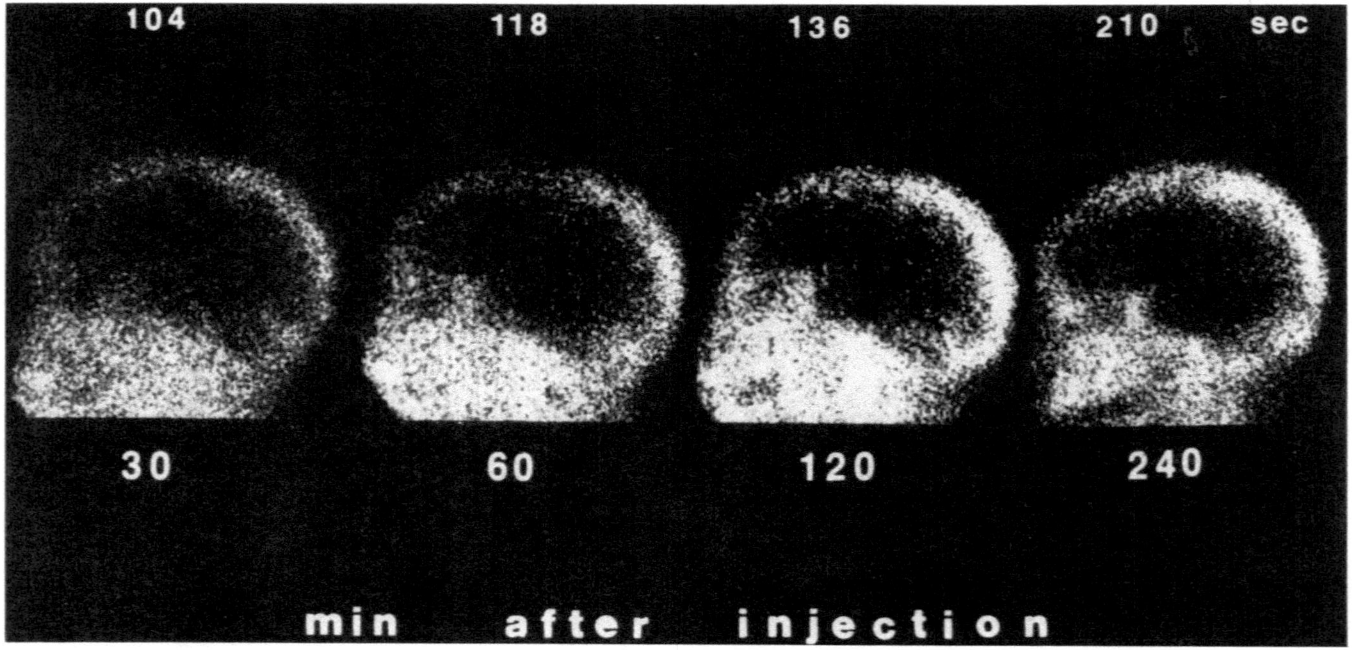

Fig. 3-2. The optimium time for collecting a ^{99m}Tc diphosphonate skull image was around 240 minutes after I.V. injection. Note the increasing length of time (seconds) required to collect the consecutive left lateral gamma camera images.

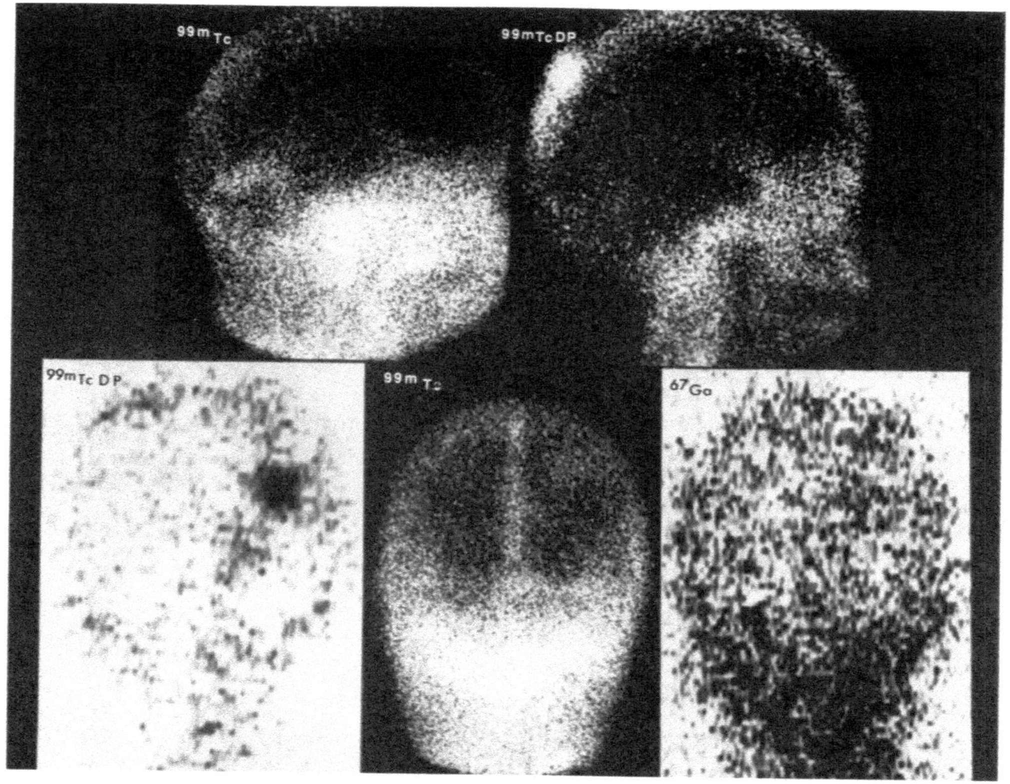

Fig. 3-3. Top: right lateral brain and skull images reveal an occipital lesion. A comparison of the 99mTc pertechnetate brain images with selected 99mTc diphosphonate gamma camera skull views will frequently provide further clarification of the rectilinear images. Bottom: from left to right, posterior rectilinear skull, posterior camera brain, and a posterior rectilinear 67Ga head view of the same patient seen in the top row.

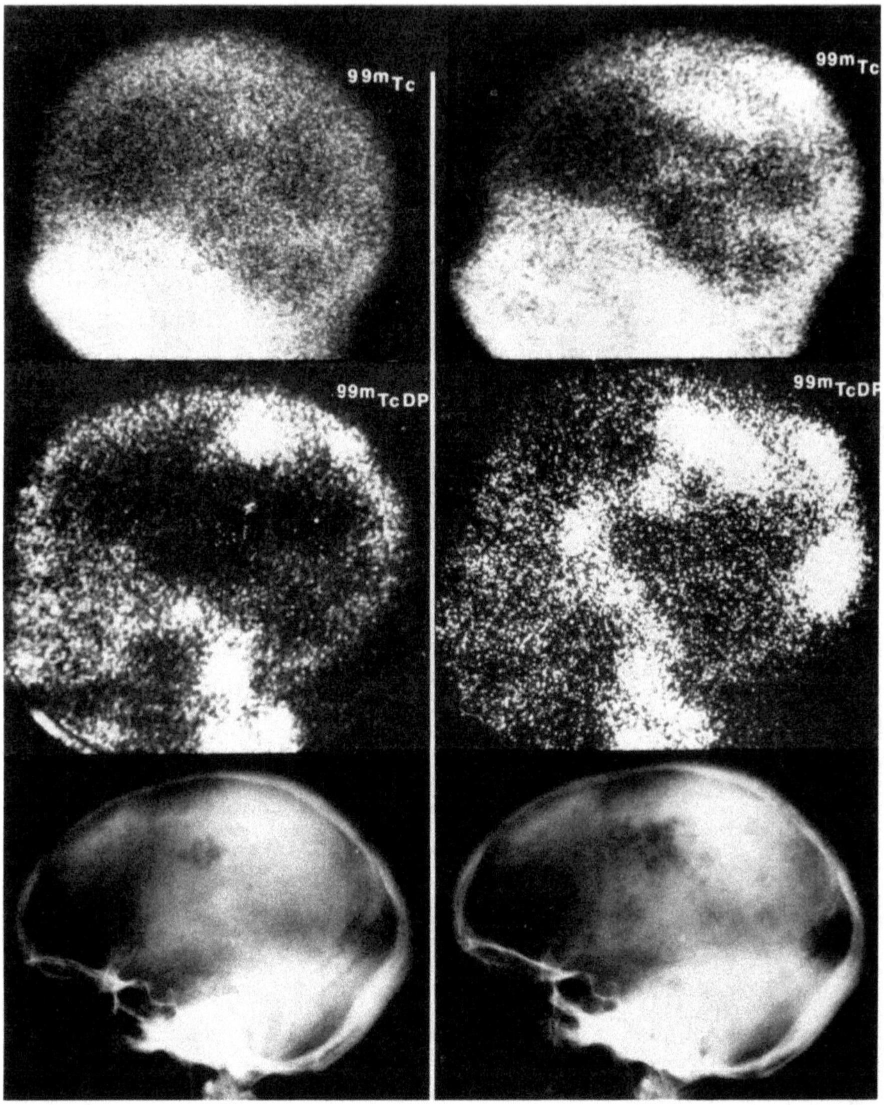

Fig. 3-4. Top: 99mTc pertechnetate brain scans; middle: 99mTc diphosphonate skull views; bottom: lateral skull x-rays. All views on the right were obtained 12 months following those on the left. The abnormalities seen on brain scan were clarified by the bone scan and lateral skull x-rays. Serial studies show the progress of the metastases. The 99mTc diphosphonate skull views defined the full extent of the lesions that are seen on the skull x-rays.

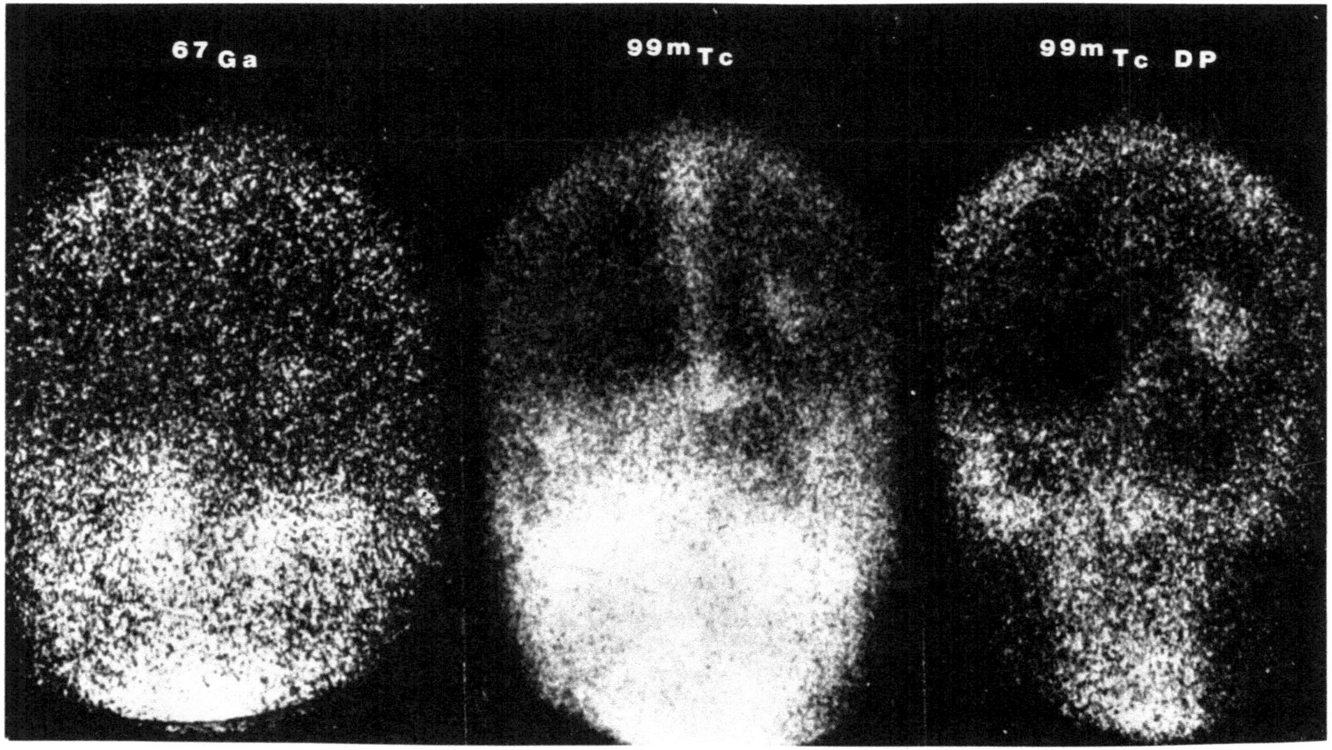

Fig. 3-5. Posterior gamma camera views left to right: 57Ga, 99mTc pertechnetate; 99mTc diphosphonate. The bony lesion was visualized in all three studies but most clearly with 99mTc diphosphonate. (Compare with Figs. 3-1 and 7 which show intracerebral breast carcinoma metastases).

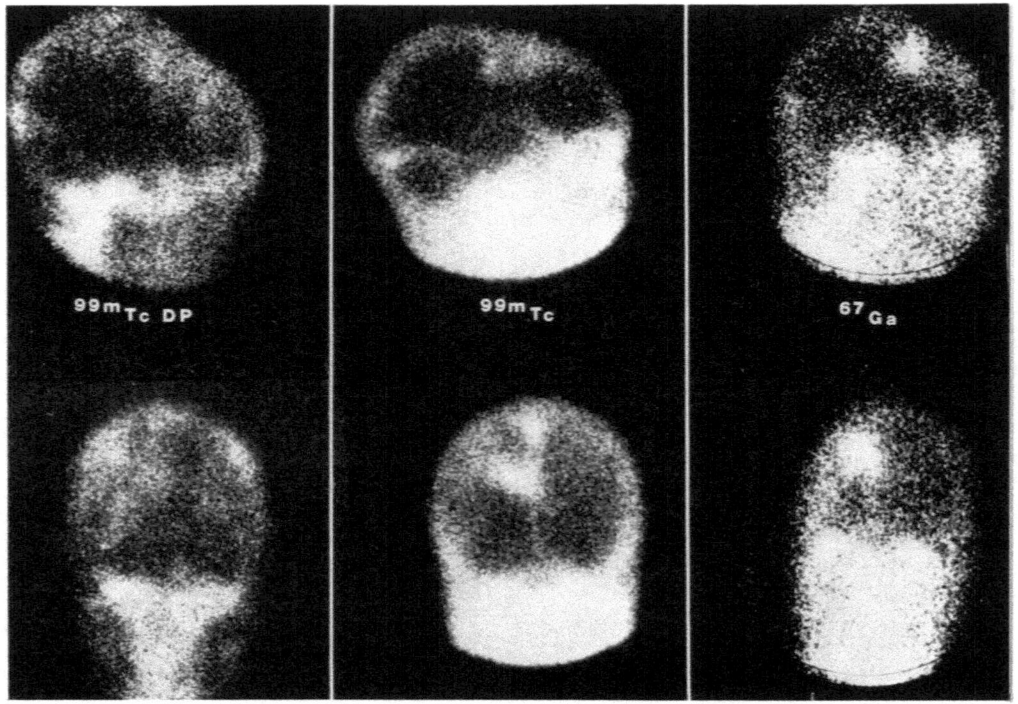

Fig. 3-6. Comparative right lateral (top) and anterior (bottom) gamma camera views of metastatic breast carcinoma. Note the extensive bony involvement seen with diphosphonate. The 67Ga selectively localized within an area suggesting a discrete tumoral component located within the defect seen on the pertechnetate brain images. The patient was known to have an extension of breast carcinoma involving the right cerebral hemisphere with a resulting left hemiparesis.

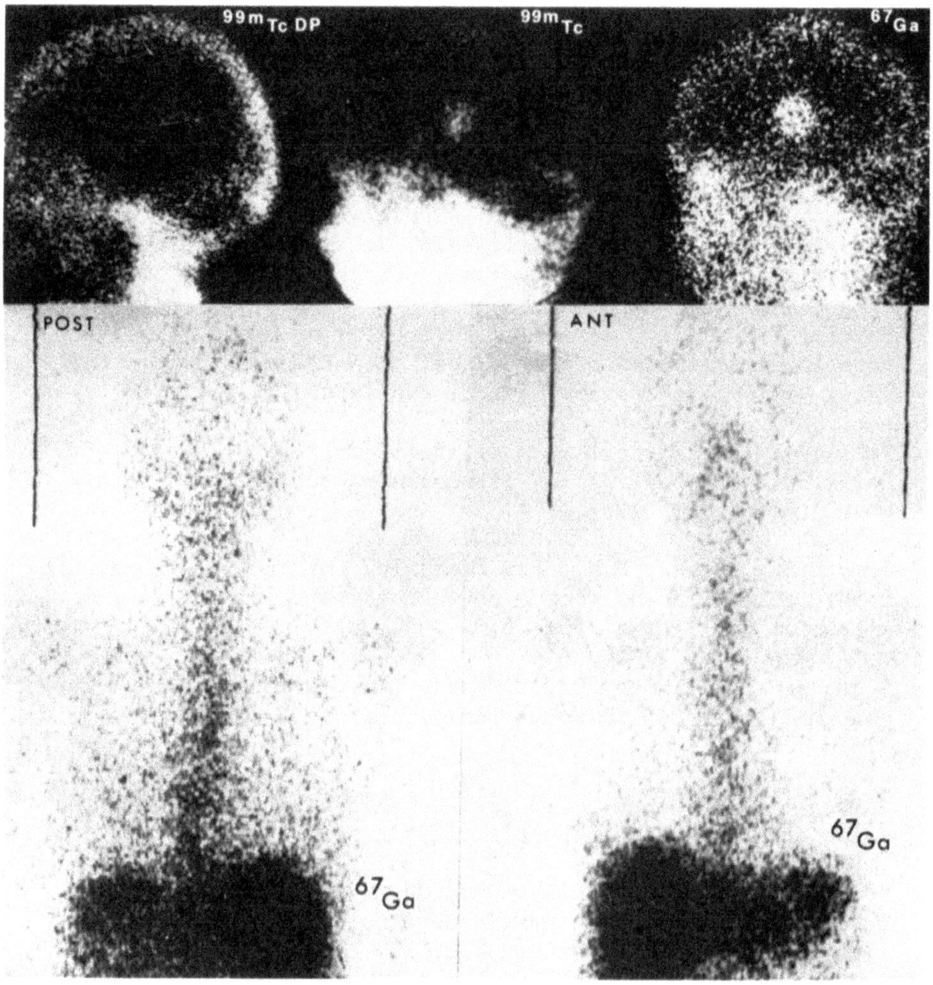

Fig. 3-7: Top row: An intracerebral breast carcinoma metastasis was clearly seen on both the 99mTc pertechnetate and 67Ga gamma camera views but was not visible with 99mTc diphosphonate. As seen in Fig. 3-6, the soft tissue tumoral component is clearly visible with 67Ga as opposed to lesions of the bony calvarium which are poorly detected with 67Ga (Fig. 3-5) Bottom: The same lesion is inadequately visualized in the posterior (left) and anterior (right) rectilinear images.

References Chapter 3

1. Brennan, M.J. Breast Cancer. In Cancer Medicine. Edited by J.F. Holland and E. Frei III, Philadelphia, Lea and Febiger p. 1769, 1973.

2. Viadana, E., Bross, I.D.J., Pickren, J.W. An autopsy study of some routes of dissemination of cancer of the breast. Br J Cancer 27: 336, 1973.

3. Abrams, H.L., Spiro, R., Goldstein, N. Metastases in carcinoma. Analysis of 1000 autopsied cases. Cancer 3: 74, 1950.

4. Haynie, T.P., III, Radionuclide imaging of brain, liver and bone in disseminated breast cancer. In Breast Cancer - Early and Late. Chicago, Yearbook Medical Publishers, p. 301, 1970.

5. Whitley, J.E., Witcofski, R.L., Bolliger, T.T., Maynard, C.D. Tc99m in the visualization of neoplasms outside the brain. Amer J Roent 96: 706, 1966.

6. Tow, D.E., Wagner, H.N., Jr. Scanning for tumors of brain and bone: comparison of sodium pertechnetate Tc99m and ionic strontium 87m. JAMA 199: 610, 1967.

7. Grames, G.M., Jansen, C., Carlsen, E.N., Davidson, T.R. The abnormal bone scan in intracranial lesions. Radiol 115: 129, 1975.

8. Maynard, C.D., Hanner, T.G., Witcofski, R.L. Positive brain scans due to lesions of the skull. Arch Neurol 18: 93, 1968.

9. Jones, A.E., Frankel, R.S., DiChiro, G., Johnston, G.S. Brain scintigraphy with 99mTc pertechnetate, 99mTc polyphosphate and 67Ga Citrate. Radiol 112: 123, 1974.

10. Meisel, S-B., Izenstark, J.L., Siemsen, J.K. Comparison of early and delayed technetium and mercury brain scanning. Radiol 109: 117, 1973.

11. Russell, D.S., Rubinstein, L.J., Lunsden, C.E. Pathology of Tumors of The Nervous System. Baltimore, The Williams and Wilkens Co., p. 225, 1963.

CHAPTER 4

Breast Scintigraphy

Steven D. Richman, M.D.

Department of Nuclear Medicine
National Institutes of Health
Bethesda, Maryland

Conventional film mammography and xeroradiography are the fundamental and most widely used techniques for the study of breast disease. Thermography is becoming established as a sensitive preliminary screening method capable of detecting early breast carcinoma. Thorough investigation with these modalities, in conjunction with clinical examination, yields greater than 90% diagnostic accuracy. Yet, equivocal cases occur all too frequently, especially in the young glandular breast. A complementary, non-invasive technique for the early detection of breast carcinoma differentiation of benign and malignant lesions has become a continuing goal in nuclear medicine.

Early attempts at isotopic breast tumor detection were relatively unrewarding. Mammary scintigraphy was initially proposed utilizing surface measurements of 32P (1) and 42K (2). Mercurial compounds have been actively studied as breast tumor scanning agents. In 1965, Sodee (3) demonstrated 197Hg-chlormerodrin localization in two of three breast carcinomas using a rectilinear scanner. Buchwald (4), using 197HgC12, studied 26 patients with this malignancy of whom 18 were positive and four were questionable. Sannazzari (5) reported nine of ten breast carcinomas visualized by rectilinear scan using 197HgC12. The high absorbed radiation dose to the kidneys with these compounds has limited their clinical application. Bonte using 131I-human serum albumin had difficulty with rectilinear image quality, as demonstrated by two fair and two poor scans in patients with large primary breast carcinomas.

The neoplastic localization of 67 Ga-citrate (67Ga) has undergone intensive clinical investigation. The affinity for 67Ga varies with the origin of the neoplasm. Primary breast carcinoma has proved less detectable than lymphoma or lung carcinoma (7)(8). Most studies, utilizing rectilinear scans, have reported suboptimal 50 to 60% detection rates for breast carcinoma.

The radiopharmaceutical most suitable for such scintigraphic study, 99mTc pertechnetate, was first proposed for extracranial tumor localization by Witley in 1966 (9). A positive finding occurred in the single breast carcinoma investigated. Cancroft (10) applied gamma camera techniques to demonstrate focal accumulation in four patients with breast carcinoma. There was no abnormal accumulation in two patients with benign breast disease. Villarreal (11) subsequently evaluated six patients with breast carcinoma demonstrating tumor localization of 99mTc pertechnetate in five. Of 30 cases with benign breast disease, six demonstrated "false positive" localization of 99mTc pertechnetate.

In a study to evaluate and compare the usefulness of 99mTc pertechnetate and 67Ga for radionuclide breast scintigraphy (12), lateral, medial and cranio-caudal gamma camera breast views were performed 15-60 minutes following the intravenous injection of 10-15 millicuries of 99mTc pertechnetate. The patient was placed in the sitting or erect position and was draped with a lead apron to allow only the breast in question to be exposed for scintigraphic study (Fig. 4-1 A,B,C). Cobalt-57 markers are placed on the collimator to note the nipple and axilla. The high resolution, low energy collimator was used for lateral and medial views; 300,000 counts were obtained with an approximate time of 200 seconds for each view. The cranio-caudal view with positioning similar to conventional mammography utilizes the pinhole collimator with a 4.5 millimeter tungsten insert. Satisafctory images are obtained in 250 seconds with 50-80 thousand counts.

Gallium-67 (50uCi/Kg of body weight) breast scans were obtained 48 hours after intravenous administration. Lateral and medial views were identical in positioning and shielding with those of 99mTc pertechnetate breast scintigraphy. The high energy collimator was used to accumulate 50,000 counts per view in approximately 300 seconds. The count rate has proved inadequate for cranio-caudal 67Ga gamma camera breast imaging.

Sixteen cases of breast carcinoma have been evaluated with 14 demonstrating abnormal 99mTc accumulation (Table 1). Discrete, focal concentration of 99m was the most common finding. There was excellent anatomical correlation with clinical, radiographic and histologic localization of breast malignancies. Of 10 patients with proven breast carcinoma, five had positive 67Ga scans, but five failed to demonstrate abnormal concentration. When both radionuclide scintiscans were positive, lesions were better visualized with 99mTc pertechnetate. Of 17 patients

Table I

Scintigraphic Mammography In Breast Carcinoma

	Positive	Negative	Accuracy
$^{99m}TcO_4$	14	2	14/16 = 88 %
^{67}Ga	5	5	5/10 = 50 %

Table II

Scintigraphic Mammography In Benign Breast Disease

	Positive	Negative	Accuracy
$^{99m}TcO_4$	5	12	12/17 = 70 %
^{67}Ga	1	9	9/10 = 90 %

with biopsy proven benign breast disease, five had abnormal localization of 99mTc pertechnetate (Table II). Gallium-67 demonstrated one false positive in 10 cases of proven benign breast disease.

Caution is necessary in supporting the validity of 99mTc pertechnetate breast scintigraphy. The high "false-positive" rate limits the use of 99mTc pertechnetate breast scintigraphy for differential diagnosis and for screening purposes. The excellent correlation between malignancy and positive breast scintigraphy (88%) may prove useful in the preoperative documentation of the extent of disease or in the evaluation of the response to therapy. Gallium-67 scintigraphy, though, a useful corroborative study when positive, is an insensitive agent for the detection of breast carcinoma. Our attempts at gamma camera scintigraphy have not improved the diagnostic accuracy noted with rectilinear scanning.

Limitations of specificity similar to that encountered with 99mTc pertechnetate have been reported with bone imaging agents employed for tumor scanning. Berg (13) reported the incidental finding of increased 99mTc-diphosphonate uptake in primary breast carcinoma in two patients undergoing skeletal rectilinear scans. Serafini (14) obtained gamma camera images demonstrating focal accumulation of 99mTc-diphosphonate or 99mTc-polyphosphate in 82% of 17 patients with breast carcinoma. However, 36% of patients with benign breast disease had positive scans as well.

Successful breast scintigraphy for tumor detection requires more selective radionuclides than those presently available. However, because of its low radiation dose and its non-invasiveness, the concept merits further investigation.

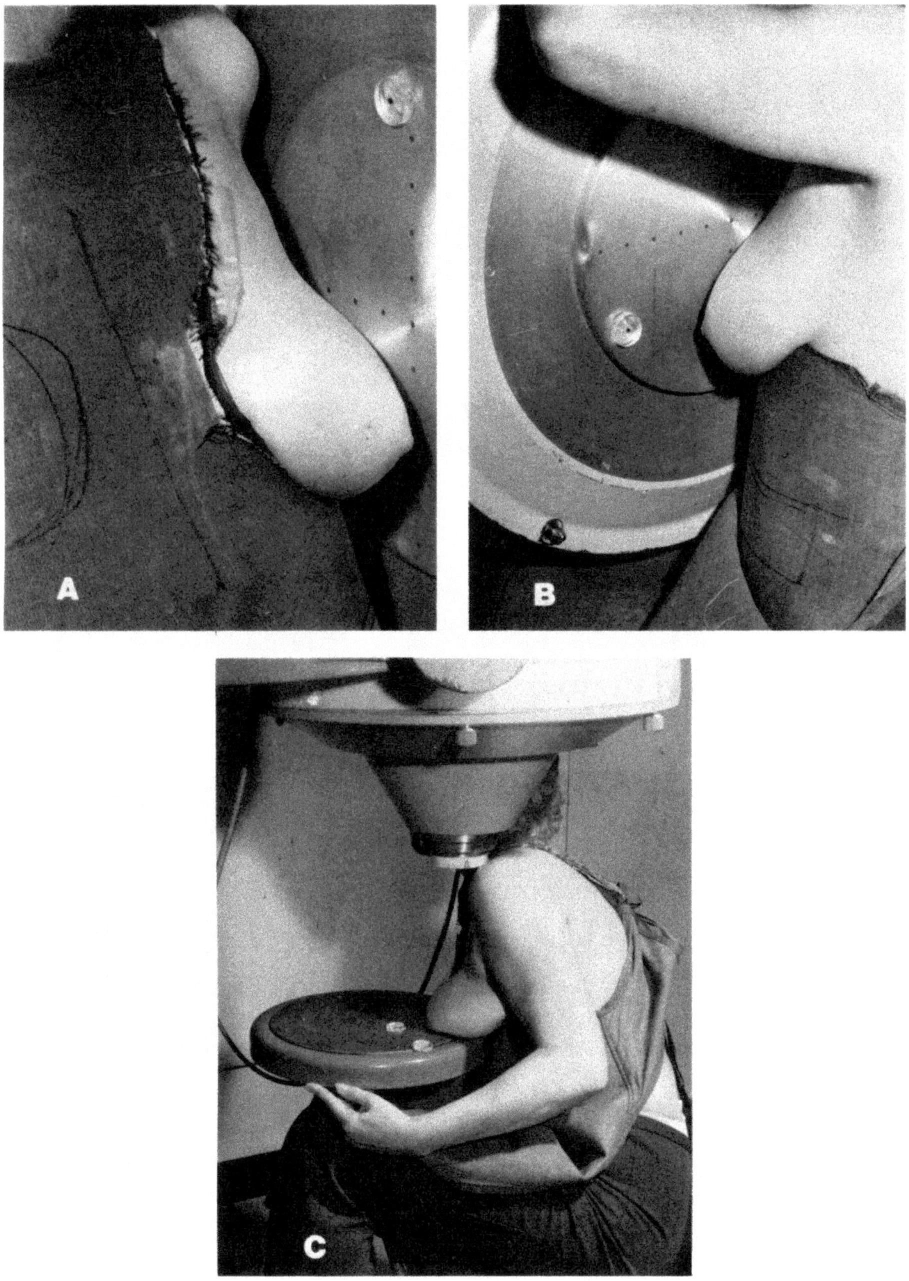

Fig. 4-1. The patient is positioned for lateral (A), medial (B), and cranio-caudal (C) gamma camera breast scintigraphy.

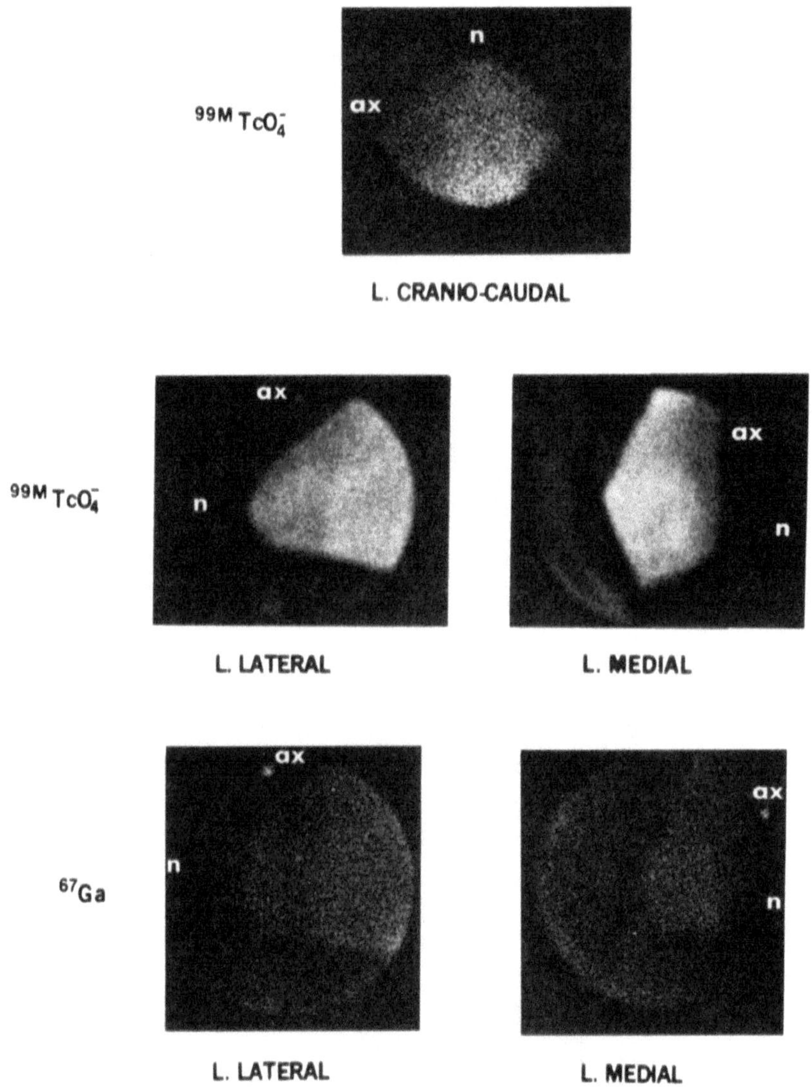

Fig. 4-2. Normal homogeneous breast scintigraphy with 99mTc pertechnetate and 67Ga citrate. There is a relative increase in radionuclide accumulation close to the chest wall in all views. The sharp delineation in the medial views is caused by the lead shielding against the chest wall. (n = nipple, ax = axilla in all of the following illustrations).

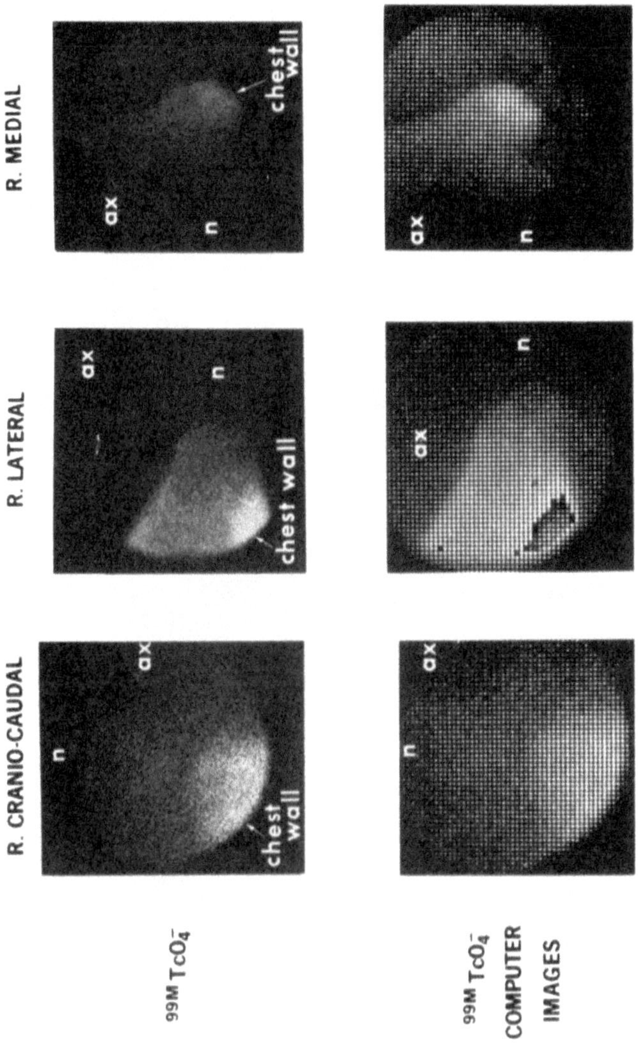

Fig. 4-3. The normal breast silhouette in 99mTc pertechnetate cranio-caudal, lateral and medial breast scintigraphy. Respective computer images are shown.

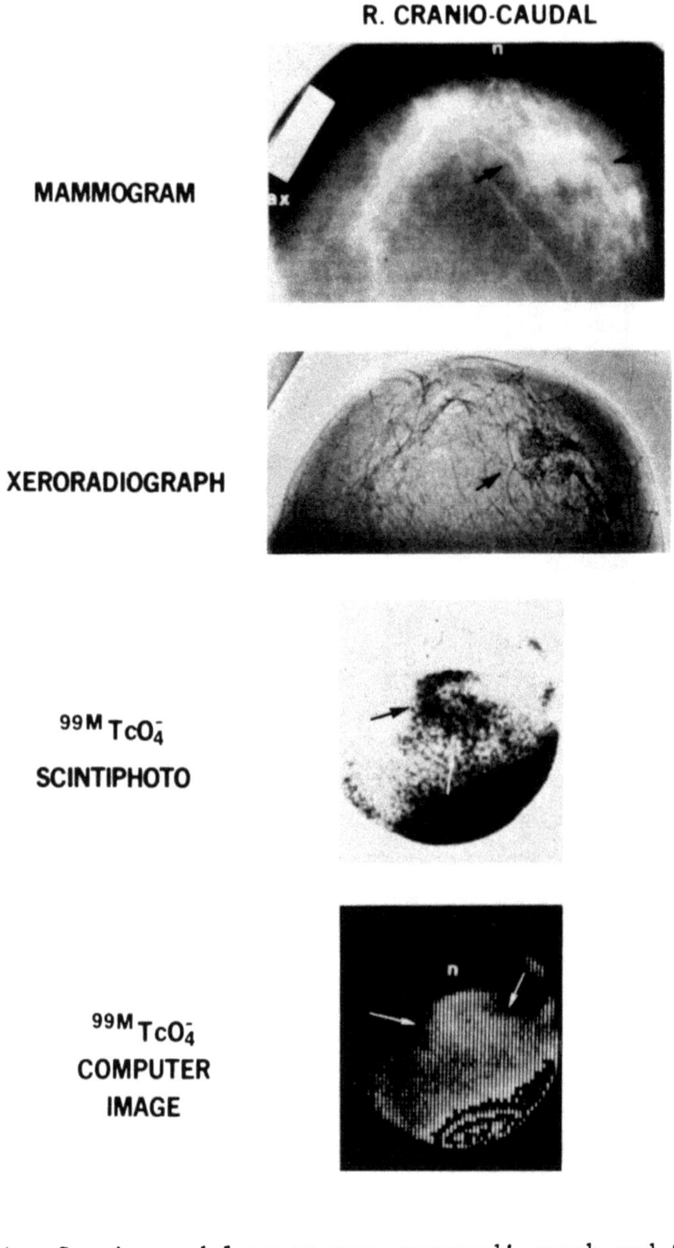

Fig. 4-4A. Cranio-caudal mammogram, xeroradiograph and 99mTc pertechnetate breast scan demonstrate a malignant mass with good anatomic correlation.

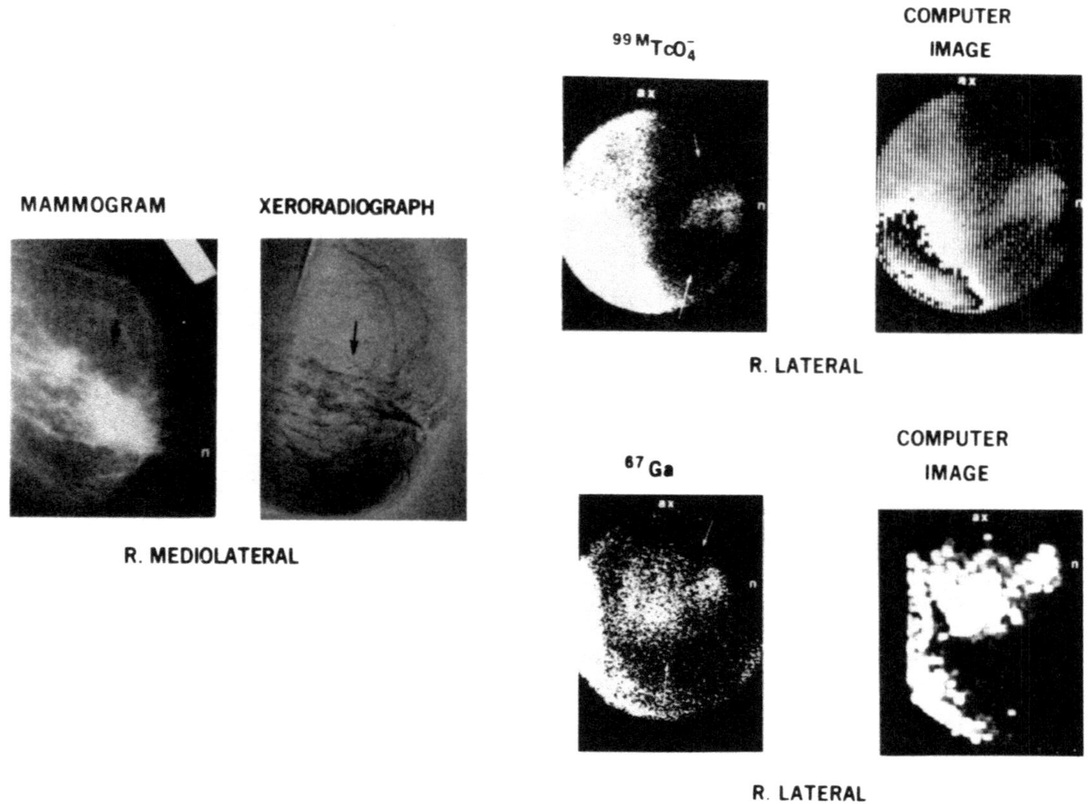

Fig. 4-4B. In the same patient, corresponding mediolateral roentgenographic studies and lateral radionuclide scintiscans show breast cancer. Computer representations can be used to confirm the abnormality.

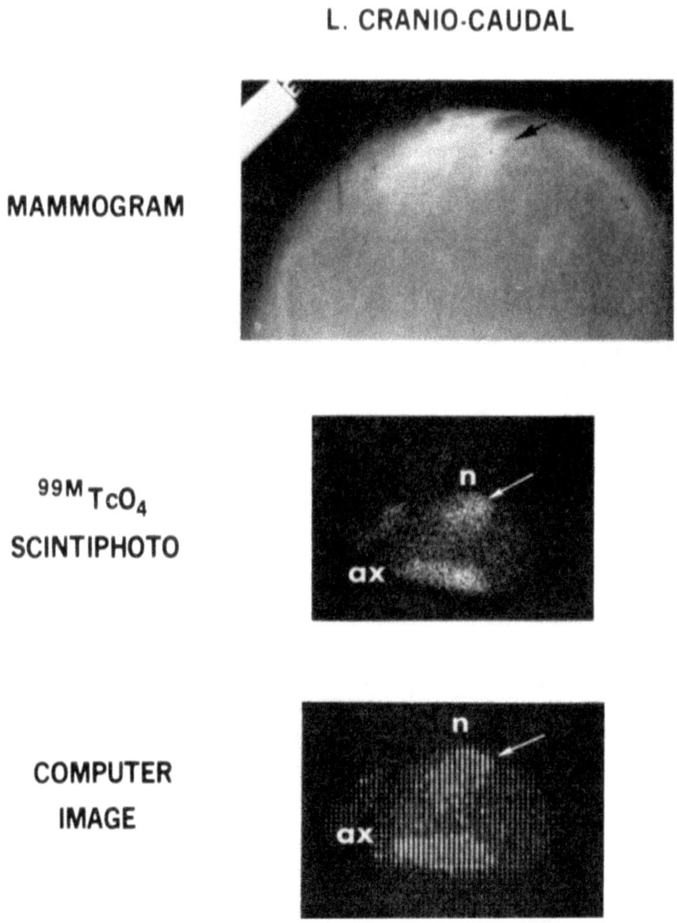

Fig. 4-5A. Cranio-caudal roentgenograph and scintiscan reveal sub-areolar breast carcinoma.

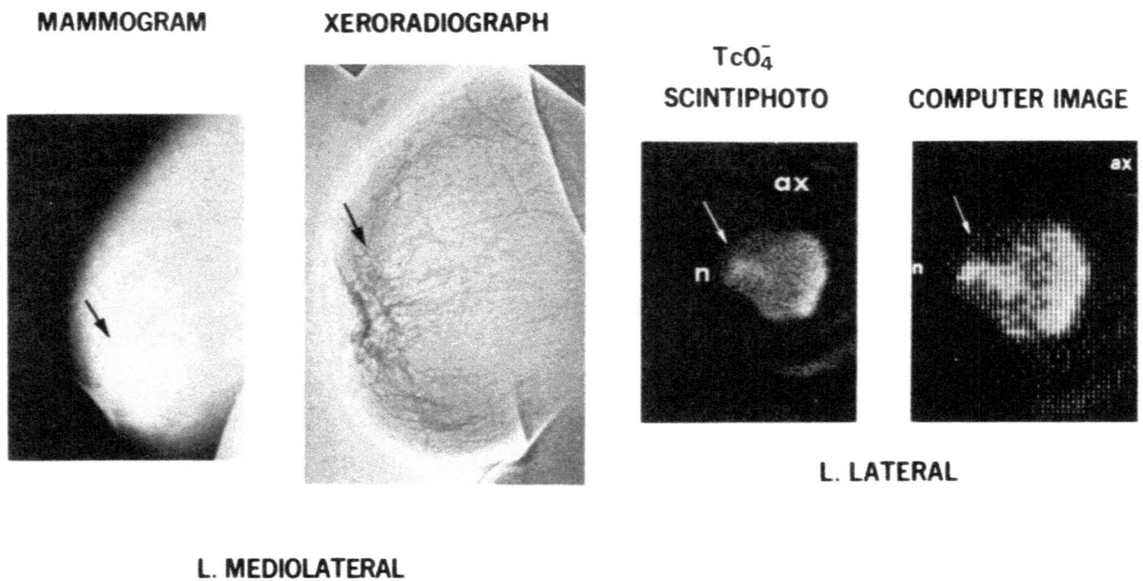

Fig. 4-5B. Mediolateral mammogram and xeroradiograph, and lateral breast scan demonstrate the same tumor. The computer image reveals a larger abnormality than previously suspected by all other means. This was confirmed at surgery.

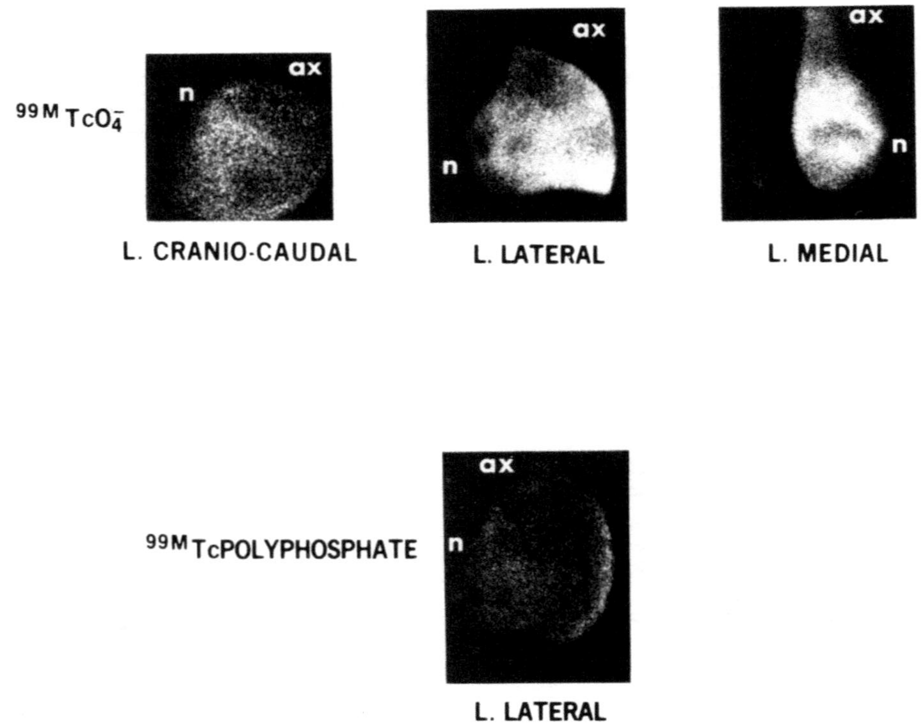

Fig. 4-6. Mottled, irregular, increased uptake of 99mTc pertechnetate followed a recent aspiration biopsy in this 48 year old woman with breast carcinoma. 99mTc polyphosphate also localized in this soft tissue tumor.

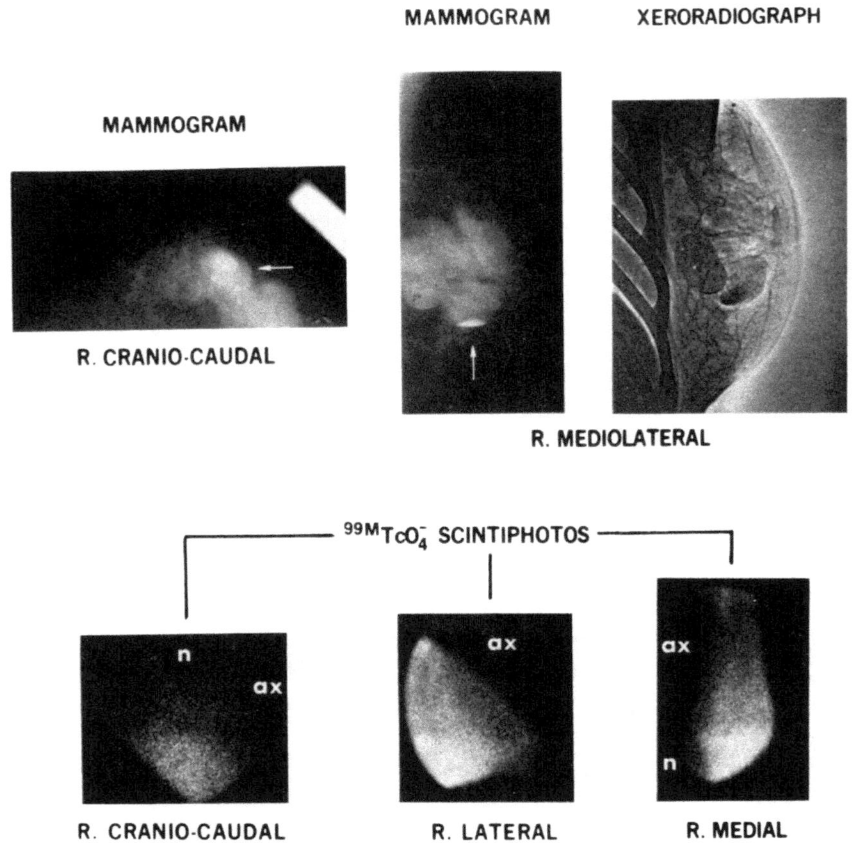

Fig. 4-7. Clinical breast evaluation in this 43 year old woman was equivocal. Large cysts with "milk of calcium" in several cysts were noted in the mammogram. Breast scintigraphy with 99mTc pertechnetate was negative and biopsy was benign.

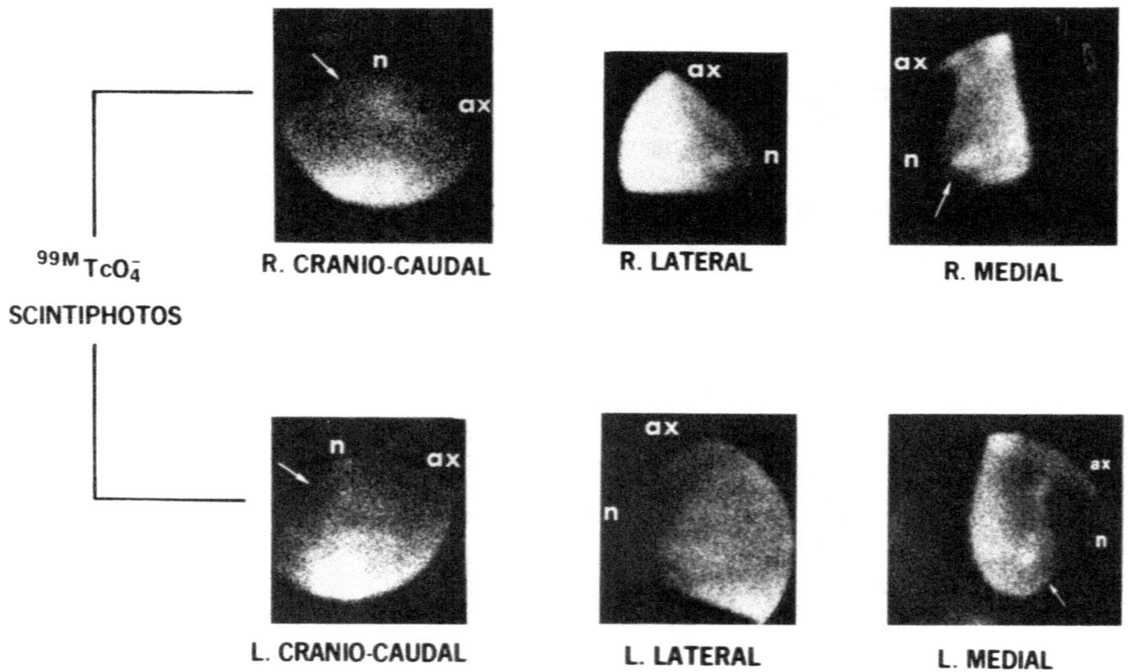

Fig. 4-8. Bilateral focal breast accumulations of 99mTc pertechnetate were noted in this patient. Abnormalities are best seen in the medial views. The left was carcinoma and a mastectomy was performed. Biopsy of the right breast demonstrated only fibrocystic disease.

References Chapter 4

1. Low-Beer, B.V.A., Bell, H.G., McCorkle, H.J. Measurement of radioactive phosphorus in breast tumors in situ: A possible diagnostic procedure; preliminary report. Radiology 47: 492, 1946.

2. Baker, H.W., Nathanson, I.T., Selverstone, B. Use of radioactive potassium (K42) in the study of benign and malignant breast tumors. New Eng J Med 252: 612, 1955.

3. Sodee, B.D., Renner, R.R., Di Stefano, B. Photoscanning localization of tumor, utilizing chlormerodrin mercury-197. Radiology 84: 873, 1965.

4. Buchwald, W., Diethelm, L., Wolf, R. Scintigraphic delineation of carcinoma of the breast and parasternal lymph nodes. In Radioactive Isotopes in the Localization of Tumors. Edited by V.R. McCready. New York, Grune and Stratton, p. 138, 1969.

5. Sanazzari, G.L., Comino, E., Negri, G.L., Baracchi, G. Radiographic and scintigraphic study of normal and pathologic breast. Minerva Med 63: 1532, 1972.

6. Bonte, F.J., Curry, T.S. III, Oelze, R.E., Greenberg, A.J. Radioisotope scanning of tumors. Am J Roentgenol Radium Ther Nucl Med 100: 801, 1967.

7. Hayes, R.L., Edwards, C.L. New applications of tumor localizing radiopharmaceuticals. IAEA Symposium on Medical Radioisotope Scintigraphy. IAEA, Vienna, 2: 531, 1973.

8. Edwards, C.L., Hayes, R.L. Localization of tumors with radioisotopes. In Clinical Uses of Radionuclides: Critical Comparison with Other Techniques. Oak Ridge, Tennessee, p. 618, 1971.

9. Whitley, J.E., Witcofski, R.L., Bolliger, T.T., Maynard, C.D. 99mTc in the visualization of neoplasms outside the brain. Am J Roentgenol Radium Ther Nucl Med 96: 706, 1966.

10. Cancroft, E.T., Goldsmith, S.J. 99mTc pertechnetate scintigraphy as an aid in the diagnosis of breast masses. Radiology 106: 441, 1973.

11. Villarreal, R.L., Parkey, R.W., Bonte, F.J. Experimental pertechnetate mammography. Radiology 111: 657, 1974.

12. Richman, S.D., Brodey, P.A., Frankel, R.S., De Moss, E.V., Tormey D.C., Johnston, G.S. Breast scintigraphy 99mTc pertechnetate and 67Ga citrate. J Nucl Med 16: 293, 1975.

13. Berg, G.R., Kalisher, L., Osmond, J.D., Pendergrass, H.P., Potsaid, M.S. 99mTc diphosphonate concentration in primary breast carcinoma. Radiology 109: 393, 1973.

14. Serafini, A. M., Raskin, M.M., Zand, L.C., Watson, D.D. Radionuclide breast scanning in carcinoma of the breast. J Nuc Med 15: 1149, 1974.

CHAPTER 5

Skeletal Scintigraphy

Robert S. Frankel, M.D.
Stanley M. Levenson, M.D.

Department of Nuclear Medicine
National Institutes of Health
Bethesda, Maryland

Since the advent of instrumentation capable of recording images of the whole body, bone scintigraphy has assumed an increasingly important role in the detection of primary and secondary bone lesions. With the recent introduction of various 99mTc phosphate bone seeking radionuclides, resultant improvement in image quality and scanning accuracy has added even more importance to this procedure in the investigation of suspected metastatic bone disease (1-5).

It is commonly felt that a metastatic bone lesion must be 50 to 70 percent demineralized before becoming visible on roentgenogram (6,7). Since localization of bone seeking radionuclides is dependent on bone turnover and regional blood flow, rather than demineralization, it is possible to detect the presence of metastases at an earlier stage than with radiographs. Numerous reports document the consistent superiority of bone scans over radiographs and clinical evidence of pain for the detection of early metastatic skeletal lesions (5-14). Charkes et al. reported 12 patients with various neoplasms in which the roentgenogram was normal and strontium-85 bone scan abnormal; biopsy or autopsy specimens from eight (67%) confirmed metastatic tumor (14). Hopkins and Kristensen correlated roentgenograms of the axial skeleton, skull and extremities with fluorine-18 and 99mTc polyphosphate bone scans in 79 patients (13). Thirty patients (38%) demonstrated lesions on the scan which were not detected roentgenographically. Metastases were confirmed by subsequent x-ray changes, biopsy, autopsy or relief of bone pain after radiotherapy. Twenty (67%) of these patients were asymptomatic.

In the National Institutes of Health breast cancer population, approximately 96% of documented or highly suspected metastatic bone lesions were present on the bone scan. Less than 3% of the metastatic bone lesions were initially detected by radiograph with a normal scan, whereas 30% of the lesions were initially detected by scan alone (15). This data is in keeping with most previously published reports (5,8,10,11).

Sklaroff and Charkes suggest that bone scans may also be of value in the early postoperative period if not performed preoperatively (11). Using strontium-85, 10 of 64 patients (15%) were found to have abnormal scans and normal roentgenograms shortly after radical mastectomy. The stage of disease at mastectomy was not defined, however all patients had "significant" preoperative adenopathy and histologically positive ipsilateral axillary lymph nodes.

Hoffman and Marty studied 47 patients with pathologic Stage I or II breast cancer within three months of radical mastectomy; 19 (40%) had abnormal strontium-87m bone scans (12). Sixteen subsequently demonstrated skeletal metastases either by biopsy, autopsy or roentgenographic changes. Roentgenograms and bone scans were compared in seven Stage I patients. Both modalities revealed abnormalities in two patients, while three patients had completely normal studies. One patient had a positive scan and negative roentgenograms, and one patient had positive roentgenograms and a negative scan. Of 18 Stage II patients, two were abnormal by both modalities, 10 were normal, and six demonstrated positive scans with negative roentgenograms.

The importance of including the bone scan in the initial diagnostic evaluation of a patient with a breast mass either suspicious for or proven as cancer, has been elaborated upon in Chapter 1. The presence of unsuspected skeletal metastases has a definite bearing on the mode of therapy (12).

Although a significant percentage of lesions are not initially present on the radiographs when detected by scan, the majority of these do appear radiographically within 2-6 months (Fig. 5-3A,B,C,). Once present on bone roentgenogram, serial radiographs are a useful way of following progression of the lesion since its size and response to therapy can be evaluated. Serial bone scans have not been particularly helpful in evaluating the activity of a lesion. In the presence of persistently abnormal skeletal scintigraphs, radiographs often reveal sclerosis in the healing stage. Although this often cannot be differentiated from sclerosis in an active osteoblastic metastasis, the changing radiographic pattern appears more useful.

The procedure of whole body bone scintigraphy consists of the intravenous administration of 10 mCi of 99mTc diphosphonate with the site of injection being recorded to avoid later misinterpretation. A three to four hour waiting period is then allowed for clearance of 99mTc diphosphonate from the soft tissues. The patient is requested to void prior to the scanning procedure in order to optimize visualization of pelvic structures.

Since those referred for whole body bone imaging had been recently studied with brain and liver scintigraphy, adequate time was allowed for the residual tracer activity to decay and clear from the patient. It was most desirable to allow a period of 48 hours to elapse. When skeletal imaging was performed first, brain and liver scintigraphy were performed the following day.

Whole body bone images were obtained with a 5 inch dual probe rectilinear scanner capable of producing 5:1 reduction images. The patient was placed in a supine position with arms and legs closely adducted and fully extended. The head was placed with the face directed upward. Following the whole body bone scan, a gamma camera view of the cervical spine was obtained with the patient's body facing into the camera and head turned sideways. All patients received right and left lateral gamma camera head views which frequently detected metastases to the cranial vault, that were either unclear or not seen on the rectilinear scans. Bilateral rectilinear cranial views, obtained as part of the whole skeletal scan, were significantly inferior to multiple gamma camera scintiphotos. This may be partially due to the patient's difficulty in maintaining a direct lateral position on the scanning table. At present however, the camera is considered the instrument of choice for cranial vault imaging. Further "spot" gamma camera views were obtained to examine other suspicious areas seen on rectilinear scan and to evaluate symptomatic regions.

Several potential pitfalls of bone scan interpretation in patients with breast carcinoma must be kept in mind. These include: contamination of clothing by urine, tracer extravation at the injection site and a contaminated alcohol sponge retained by the patient. Camera views will usually clarify these artefacts. Since benign lesions also appear as areas of increased uptake on the scan, these too must be distinguished from metastatic disease. Therefore, it is always necessary to consider the possibility of a recent fracture, benign bone tumor or Paget's disease (Fig. 5-18), before ascribing an abnormal radionuclide accumulation to metastatic disease. If such benign lesions can be reasonably ruled out by history, physical and radiographic evaluations, the accuracy of an abnormal bone scan as an indication of metastasis approaches 95%.

Soft tissue localization of bone seeking radionuclides must be recognized as such and not interpreted as skeletal in origin. Localization in the region of a recent mastectomy site can usually be differentiated from rib lesions by its diffuse rather than discrete nature of appearance (Fig. 5-11A). Accumulation of 99mTc diphosphonate has also been seen in a cancerous breast prior to its removal (Fig. 5-17), as well as in normal breast tissue. Asymmetries of 99mTc diphosphonate localization are frequently noted following mastectomy and radiation therapy; respectively, these demonstrate diffuse, unilateral thoracic increases and decreases in radioactivity (Fig. 5-6A). In other areas that have received radiotherapy, diminished 99mTc diphosphonate activity may also be noted.

Radionuclide accumulation in the skull can present interpretive difficulities since 99mTc phosphate compounds accumulate in cerebral metastases or cerebral infarcts, as well as in cranial vault metastases (17). Localization of 99mTc diphosphonate in brain lesions is often less intense and more diffuse than when it is seen in metastases to the skull (Chapter 3 Fig. 3-1 and 5).

On occasion, a patient with diffuse skeletal metastases may present with a normal appearing bone scan (5,18,19). These cases have been unusual in their clarity of bony definition. The ribs are particularly well delineated. Although there is an increased amount of radioactivity in the skeleton, the lack of asymmetries lead the viewer to falsely believe that the scan is normal (Fig. 5-15A).

Following chemotherapy, bone scan abnormalities may show an increased amount of radioactivity, or new areas may appear. These can be misconstrued as progression of disease when in fact, healing with increased osteoblastic activity is the explanation. In this situation, the differentiation of disease progression from regression is aided by knowledge of the patient's clinical status.

Since the labeled phosphate bone imaging agents are cleared by the kidneys, it is of value to observe the position, size, and intensity of renal radionuclide localization. When a significant renal asymmetry is noted, there is an 85% chance of some renal abnormality (20,21). Ureteral visualization and bladder contour should also be considered.

In summary, whole body bone scans provide information concerning the site and extent of disease in patients with primary and metastatic carcinoma. The procedure may be repeated during and following therapy in order to assess the response to treatment or to detect recurrent sites of disease. Whole body bone scintigraphy has proven an invaluable aid in the investigation of breast carcinoma metastatic to bone. Its superiority to radiographic studies in the detection of early metastatic bone lesions is well documented. As with other nuclear medical procedures, it should not be used in an isolated manner, but rather as an adjunct to other available modalities.

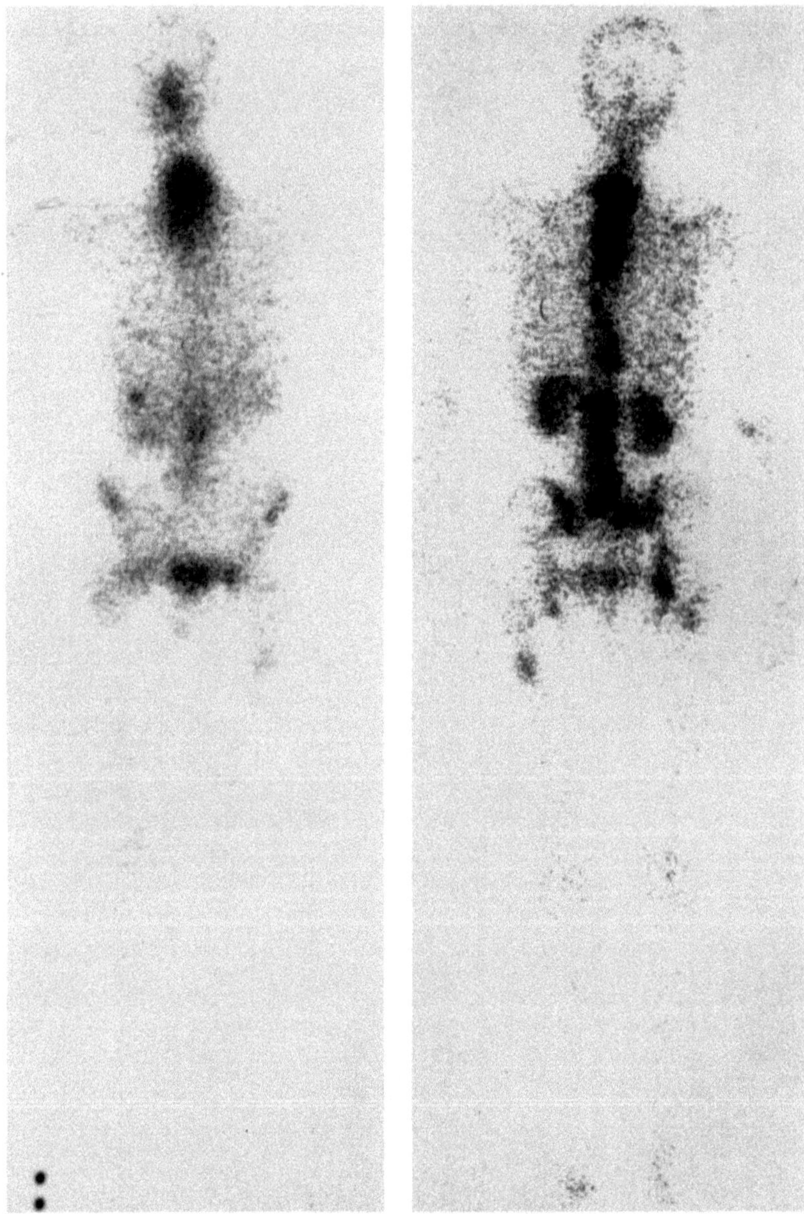

Fig. 5-1. 99mTc diphosphonate scans (anterior and posterior) show diffuse metastases evidenced by multiple areas of increased nuclide concentration in the anterior ribs, spine, sacrum, left sacroiliac joint, right ischium, right femoral head, and proximal third of the left femoral shaft. The intensity of uptake in the upper thoracic spine is so great that activity is seen to "shine through" on the anterior view. Radiographs also showed diffuse skeletal metastases.

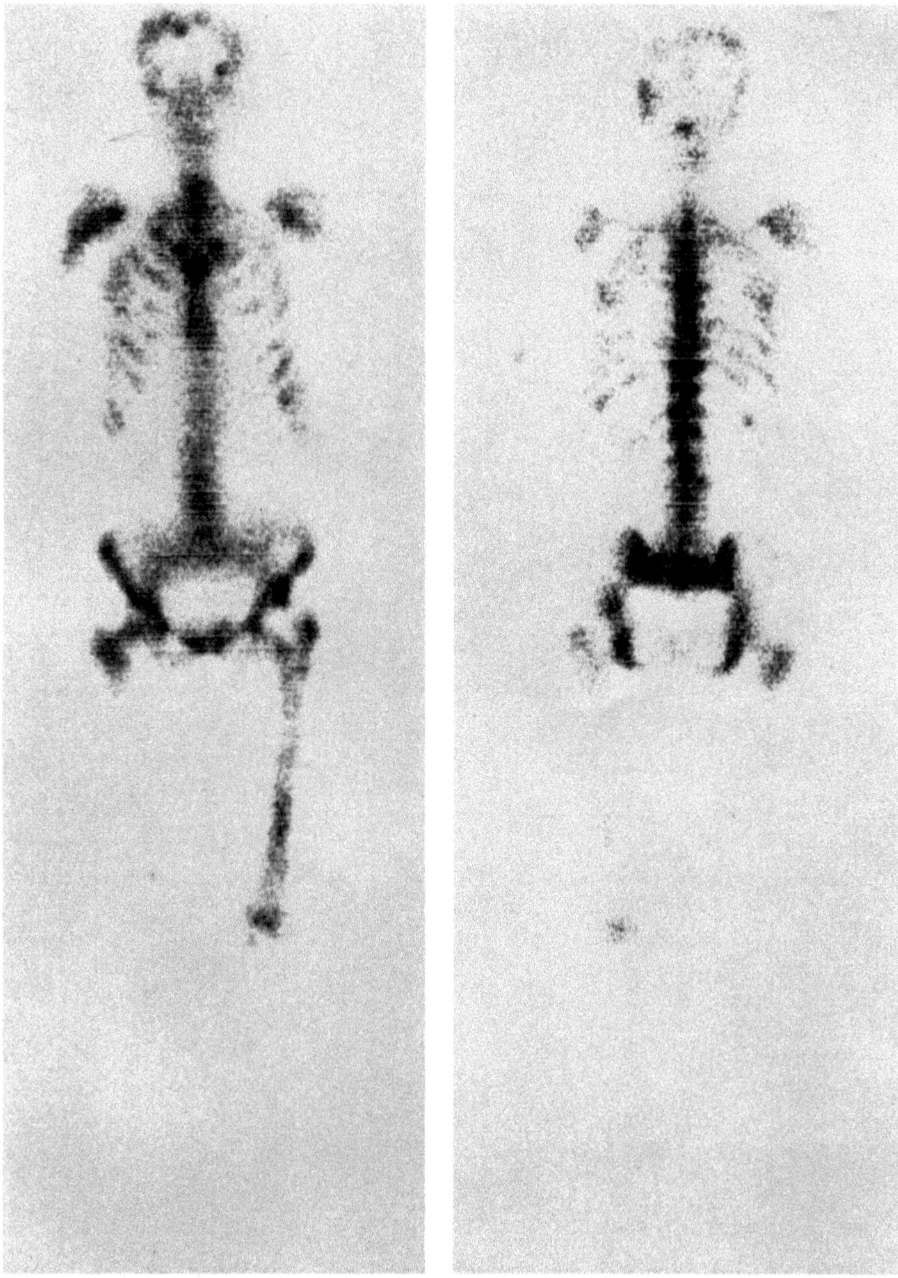

Fig. 5-2. In a patient with metastatic breast carcinoma, the 99mTc diphosphonate scans show abnormal nuclide accumulation in the skull, both shoulders, ribs, entire spine, pelvis and left femur. Radiographic skeletal survey was also abnormal but did not detect as many of the skull and rib lesions.

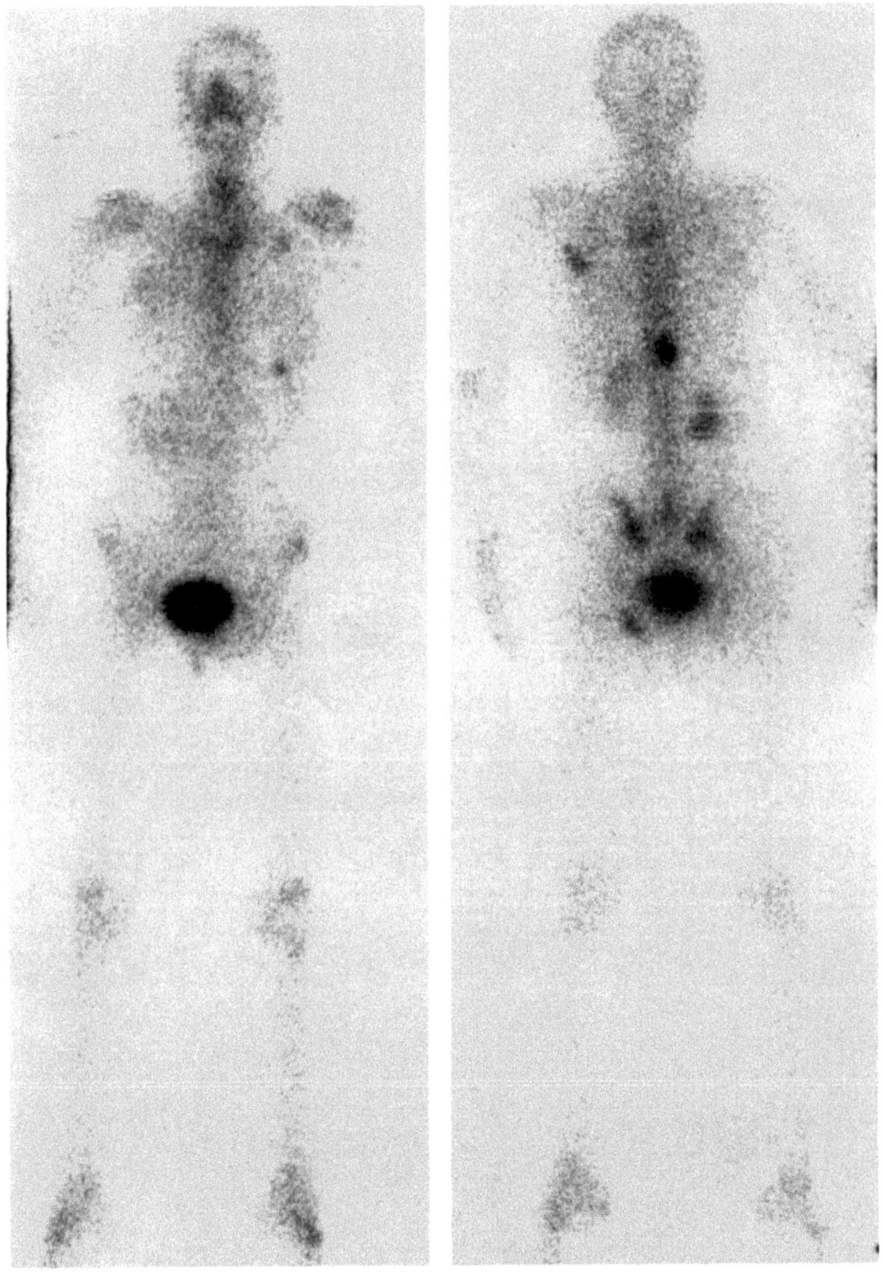

Fig. 5-3A. Anterior and posterior whole body scans with 99mTc diphosphonate show areas of increased uptake in the left anterior rib cage, left posterior rib cage or scapular tip, lower thoracic spine, lower lumbar spine, scaroiliac joints, and left ischium.

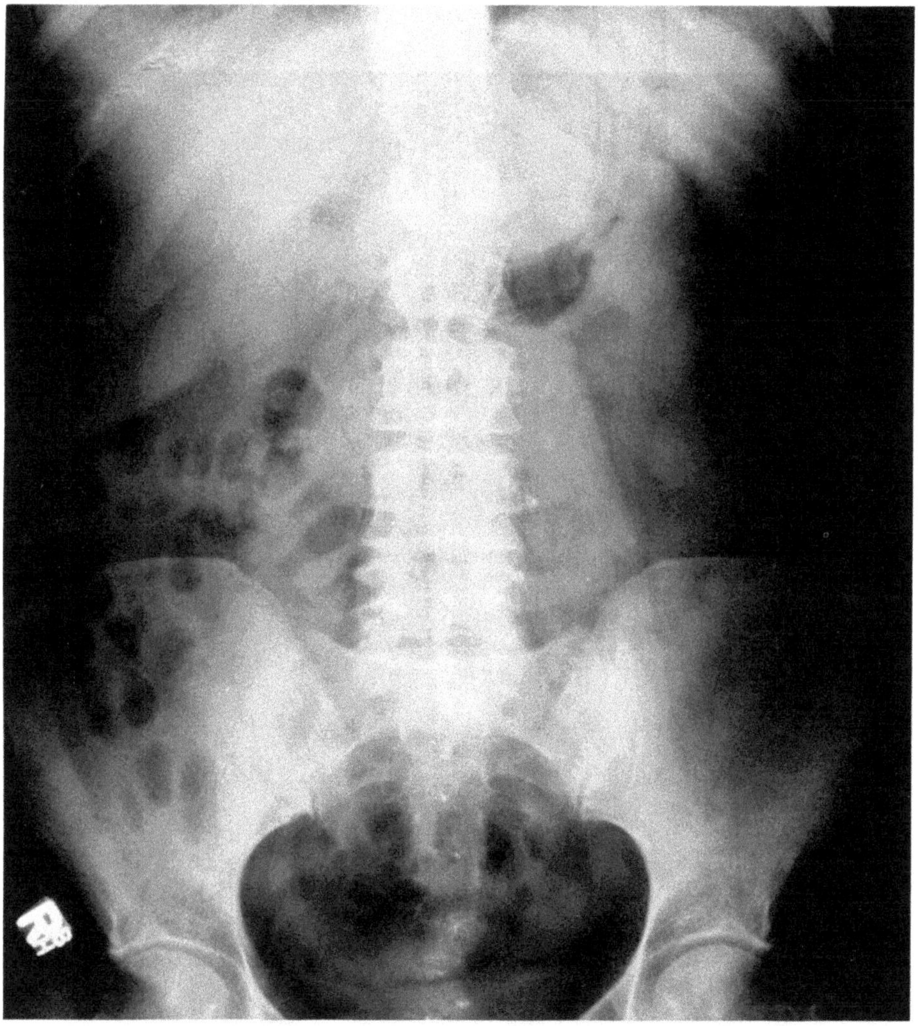

Fig. 5-3B. The only apparent metastatic lesion on the radiographic survey of this patient was in the left ischium. All other areas either became abnormal on radiographs within the ensuing nine months or became clinically symptomatic.

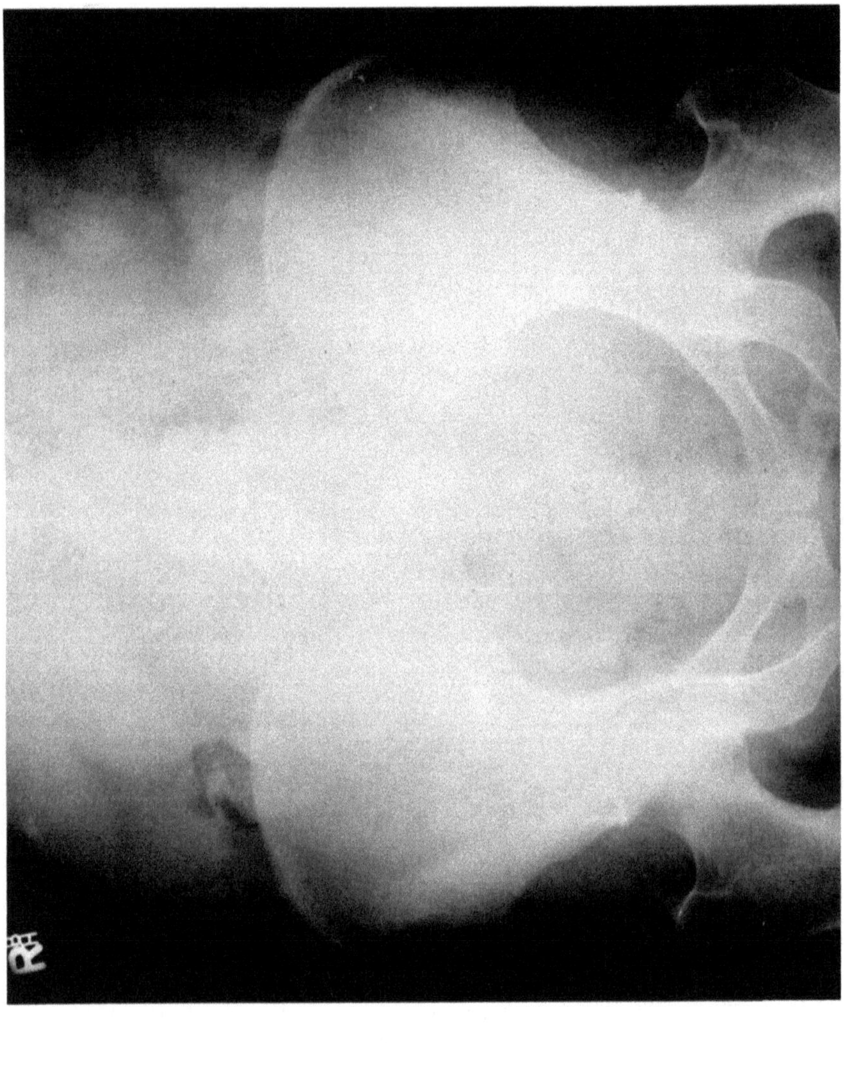

Fig. 5-3C. See caption of Fig. 5-3B.

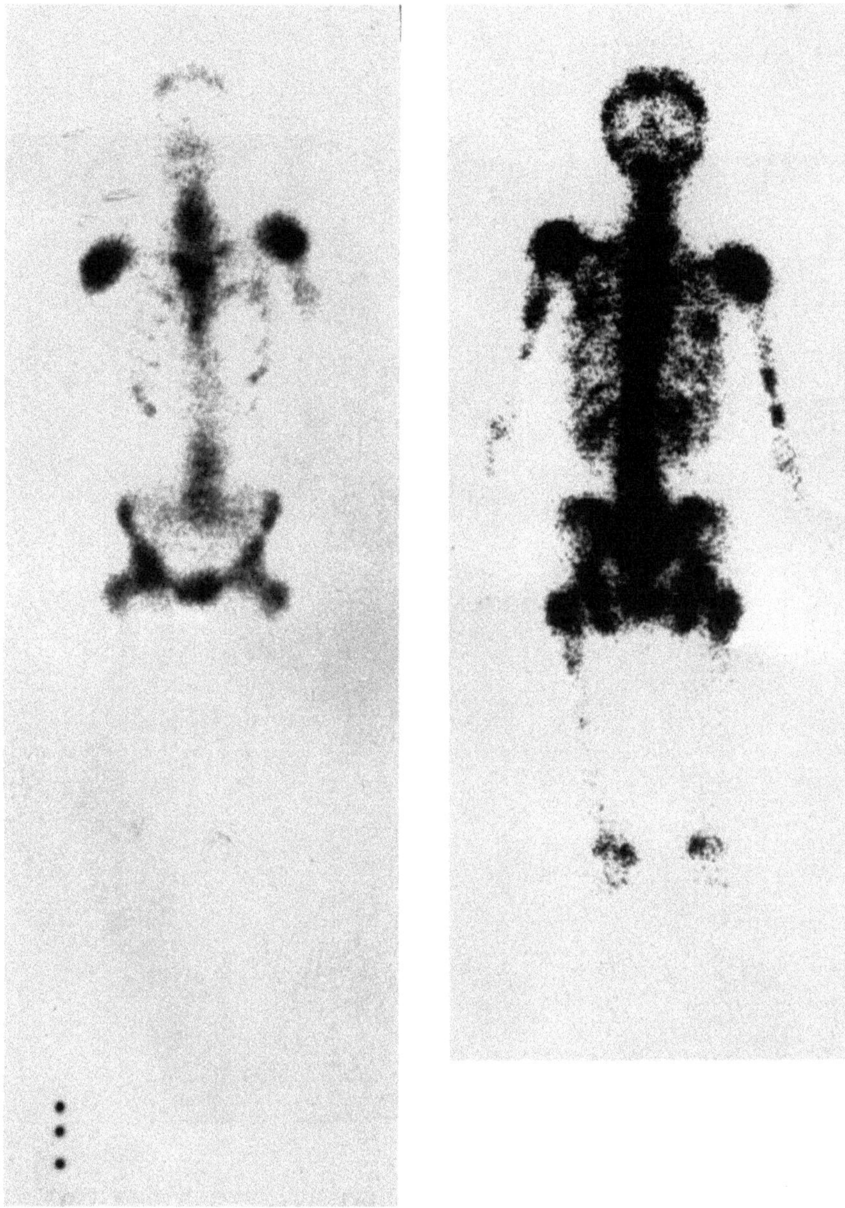

Fig. 5-4A. 99mTc diphosphonate scans on this patient with bilateral shoulder pain reveal increased nuclide accumulations in the shoulders and humeral shafts bilaterally. There is also diffusely increased uptake in the spine suggestive of diffuse metastatic involvement. Uptake throughout the pelvis is greater than normal, especially in the ischii and femoral heads bilaterally and the proximal portion of the left femoral shaft on the posterior scan.

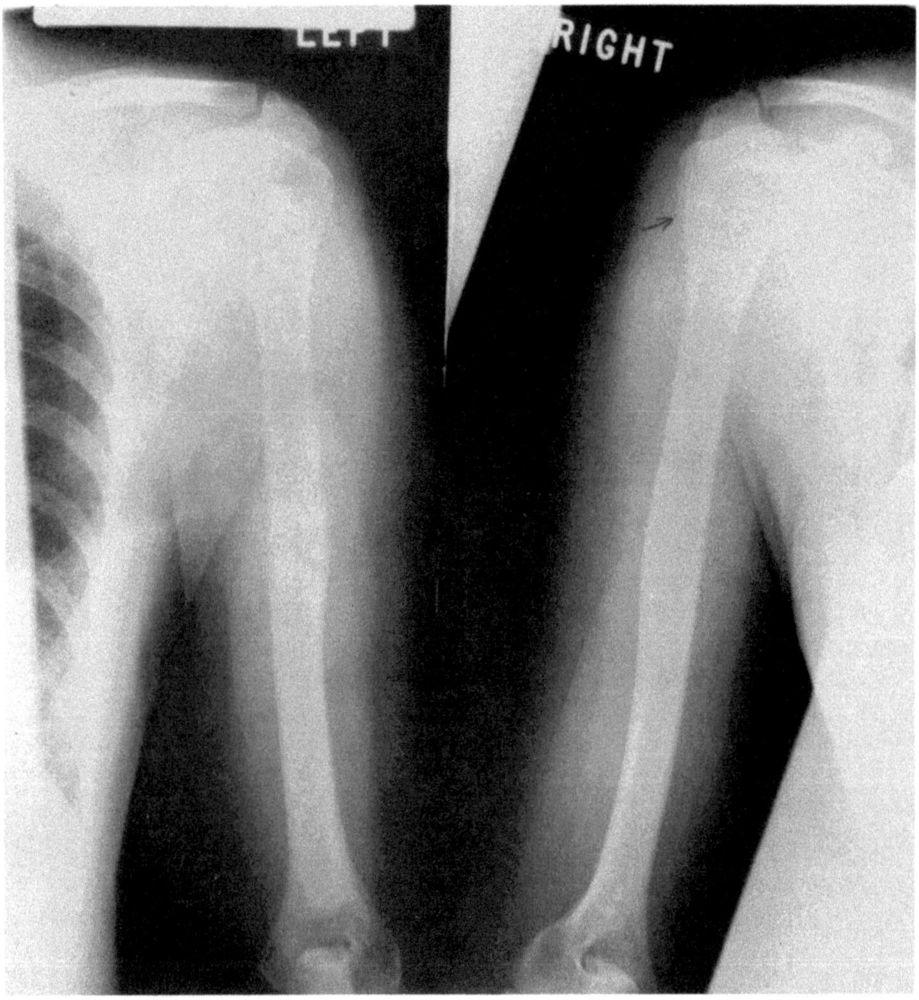

Fig. 5-4B. Radiographs of the shoulders and humeri show only minimal erosive changes in the right upper humeral shaft. Films two months later continued to be normal except for this one finding.

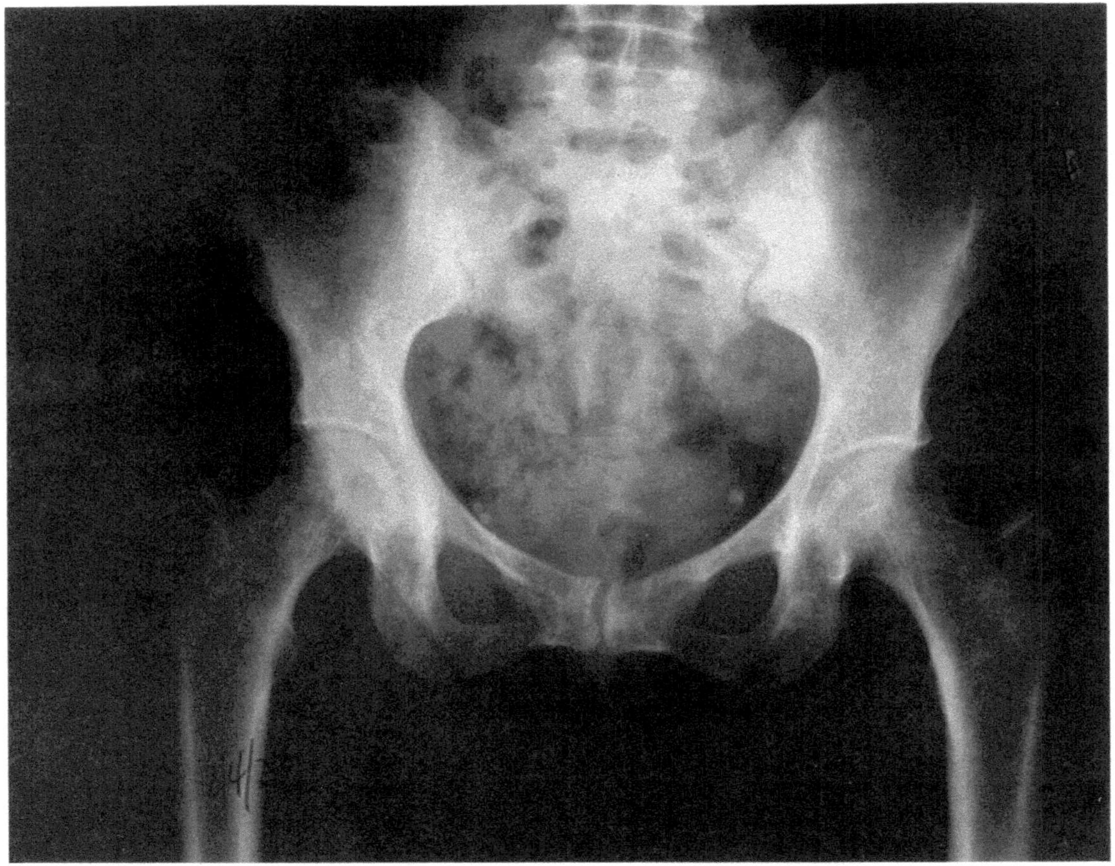

Fig. 5-4C. Radiography of the pelvis shows no definite abnormalities. Two months later, the patient developed diffuse pelvic pain with a persistent normal radiograph.

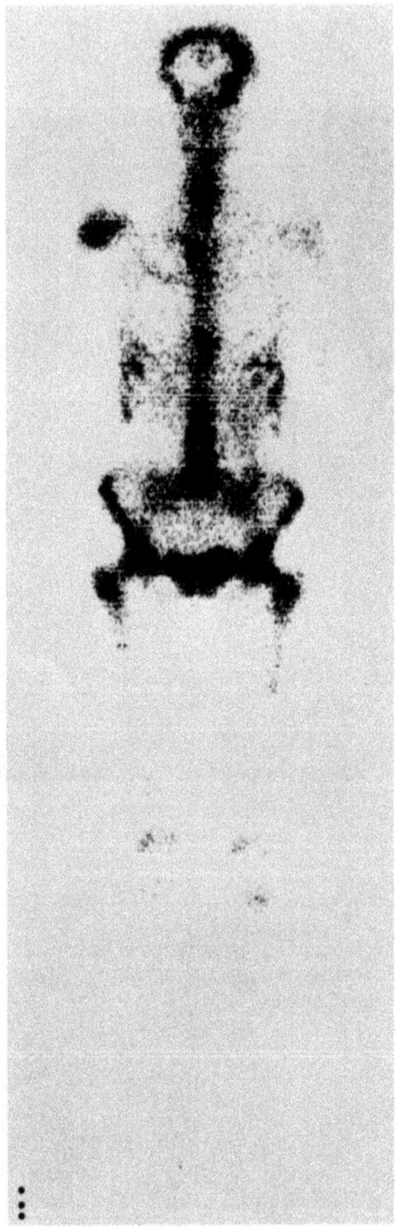

Fig. 5-5A. Anterior 99mTc diphosphonate bone image of this patient shows multiple metastatic sites including the skull, right shoulder, thoraco-lumbar spine, ribs, and much of the pelvis.

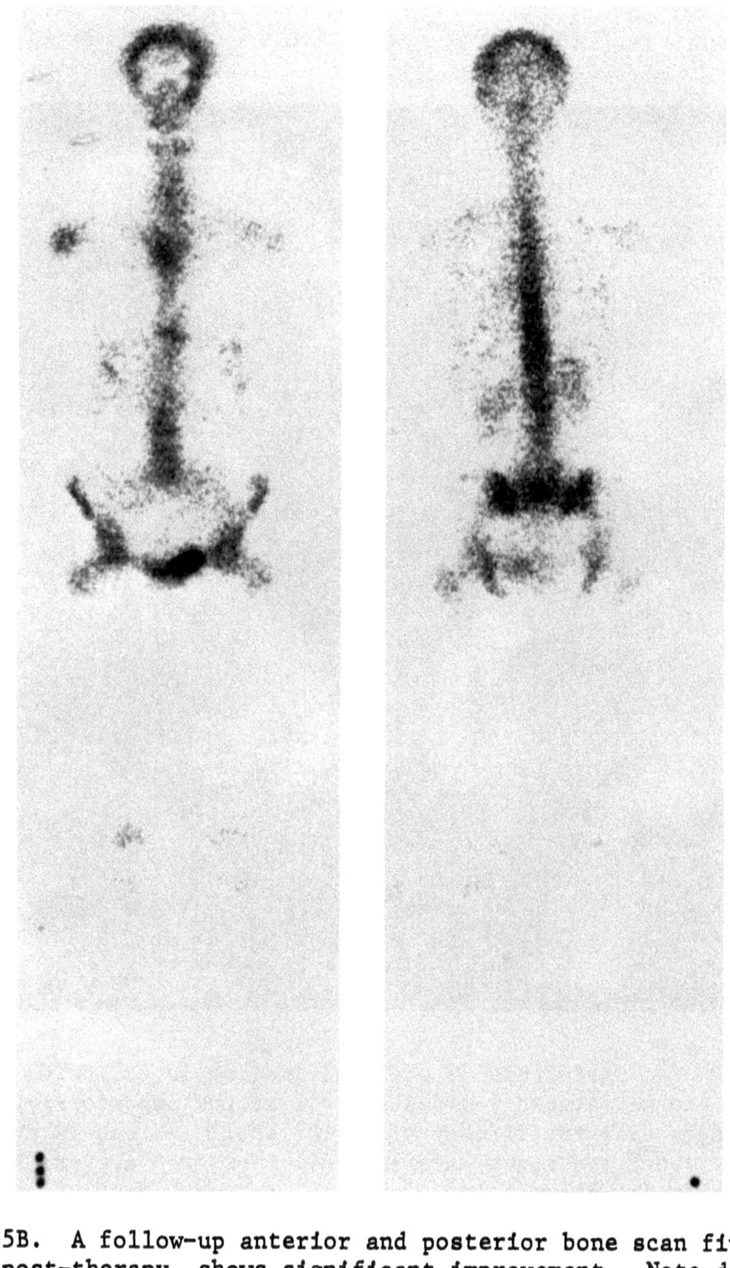

Fig. 5-5B. A follow-up anterior and posterior bone scan five months later, post-therapy, shows significant improvement. Note decreased localization of bone agent in the anterior chest bilaterally. This occurred following radiation therapy to these areas.

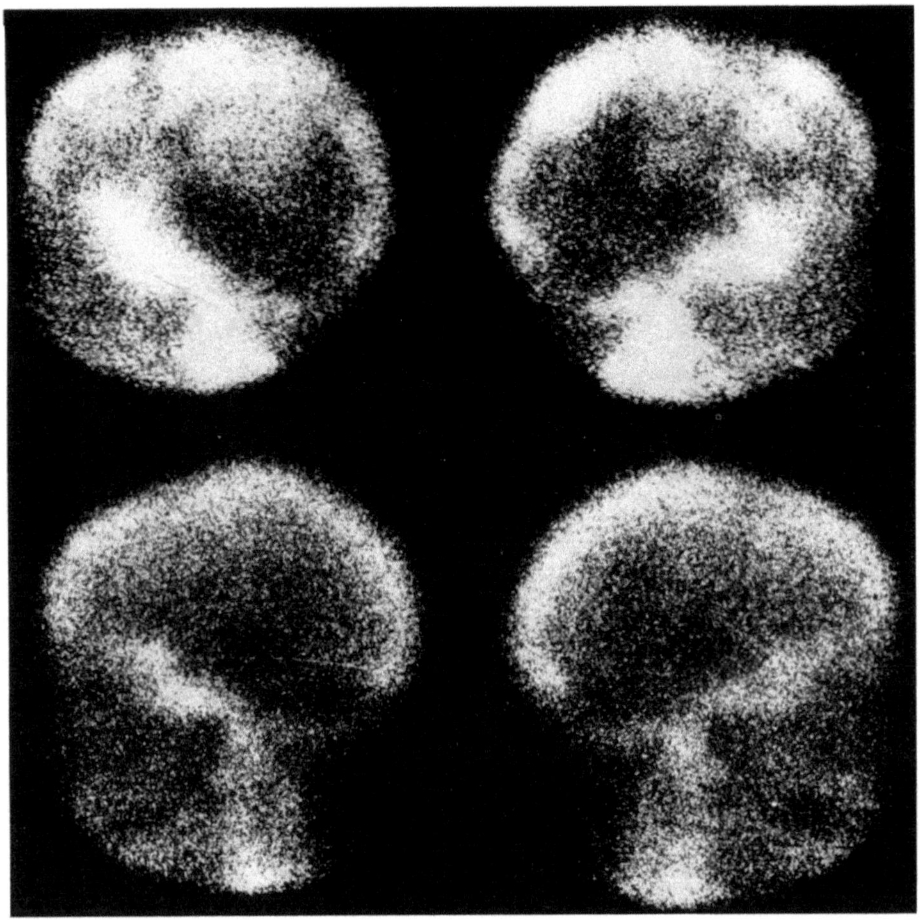

Fig. 5-5C. The usefulness of skeletal imaging in following the course of the metastatic lesions as well as the superiority of camera images over rectilinear views for skull lesions is evident in this case. Left and right lateral skull views above, were obtained prior to therapy; those below, following therapy.

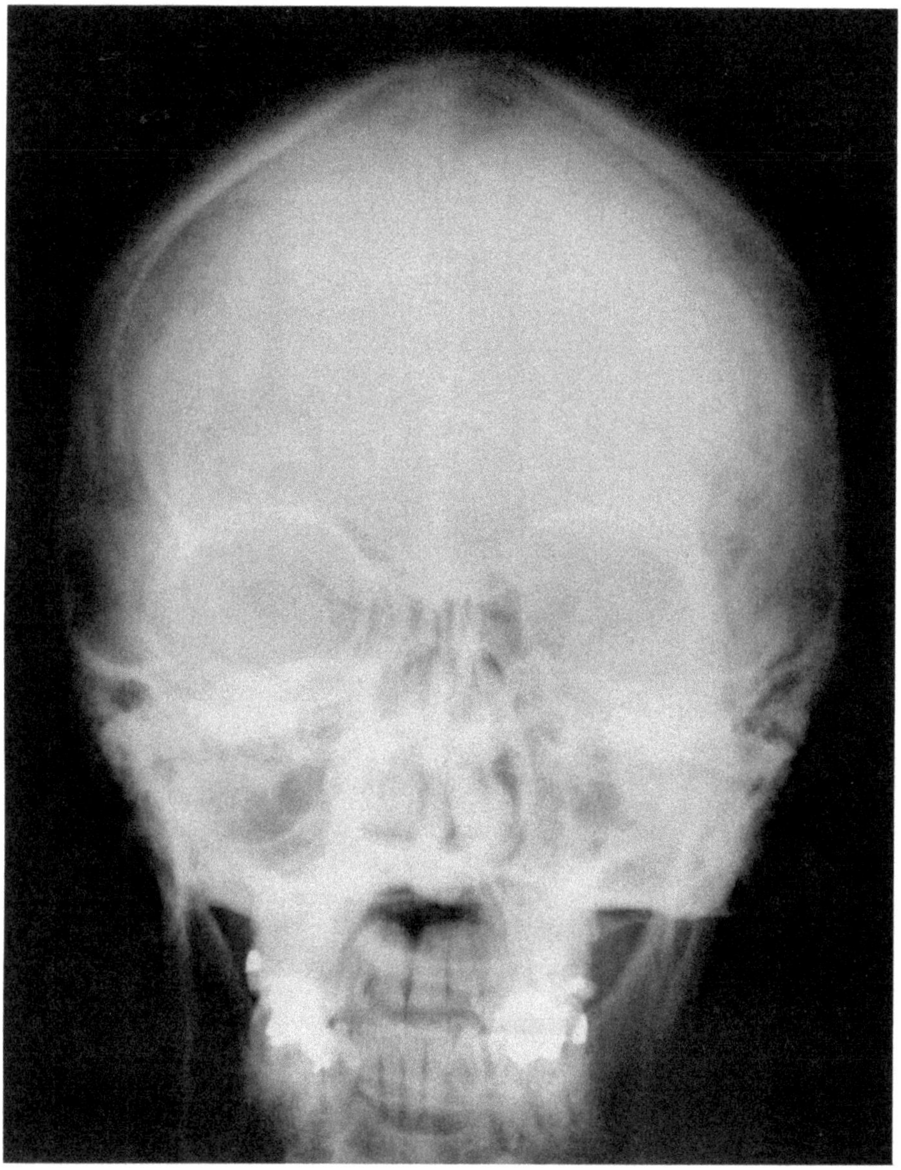

Fig. 5-5D. Skull radiographs at the time of the initial positive scan of the head, were interpreted as normal.

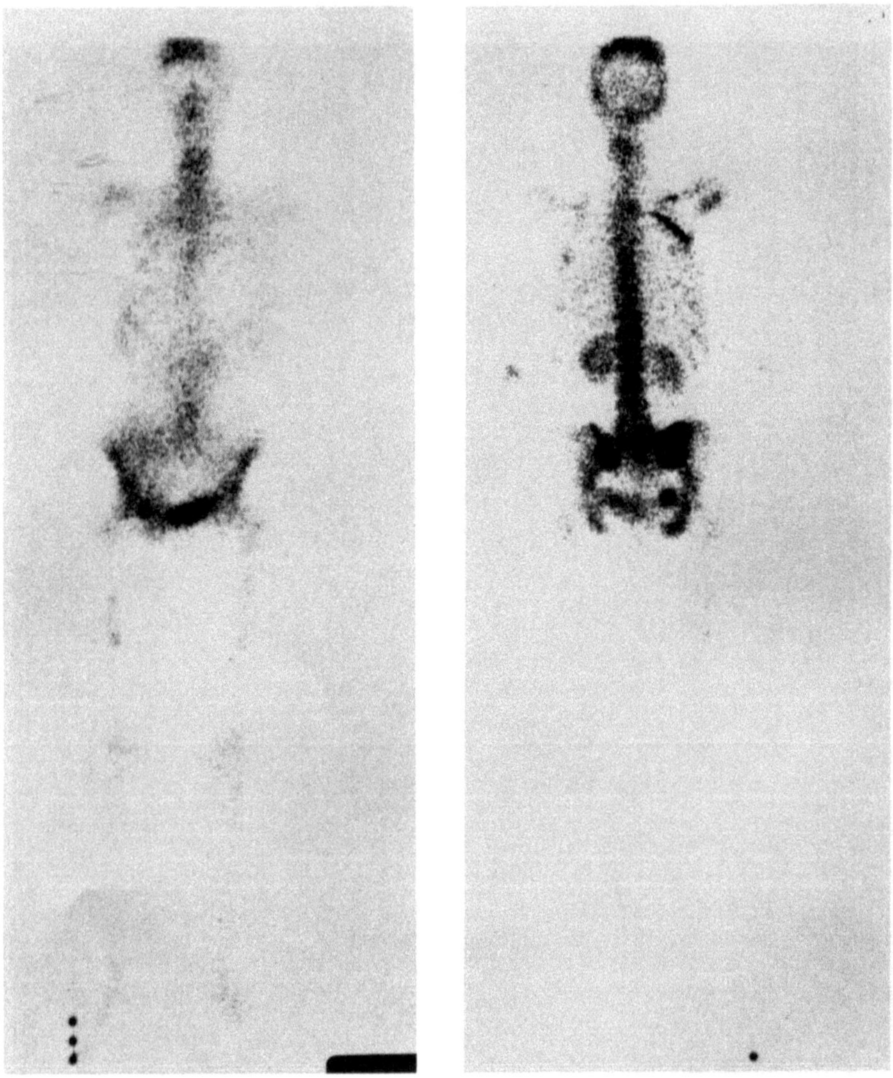

Fig. 5-6A. Anterior and posterior 99mTc diphosphonate bone scans show areas of increased uptake in the skull, S-I joints, right pubic bone and posterior right chest. This latter finding was interpreted as being either in the scapula or a posterior rib. Radiographic study revealed the lesion to be in the rib. The need for correlation with radiographic studies is important since scanning is not as anatomically specific, although more sensitive then roentgenograms. The patient had a modified left mastectomy with post operative radiation therapy. Note the decreased localization of bone agent in the left anterior chest associated with radiation therapy.

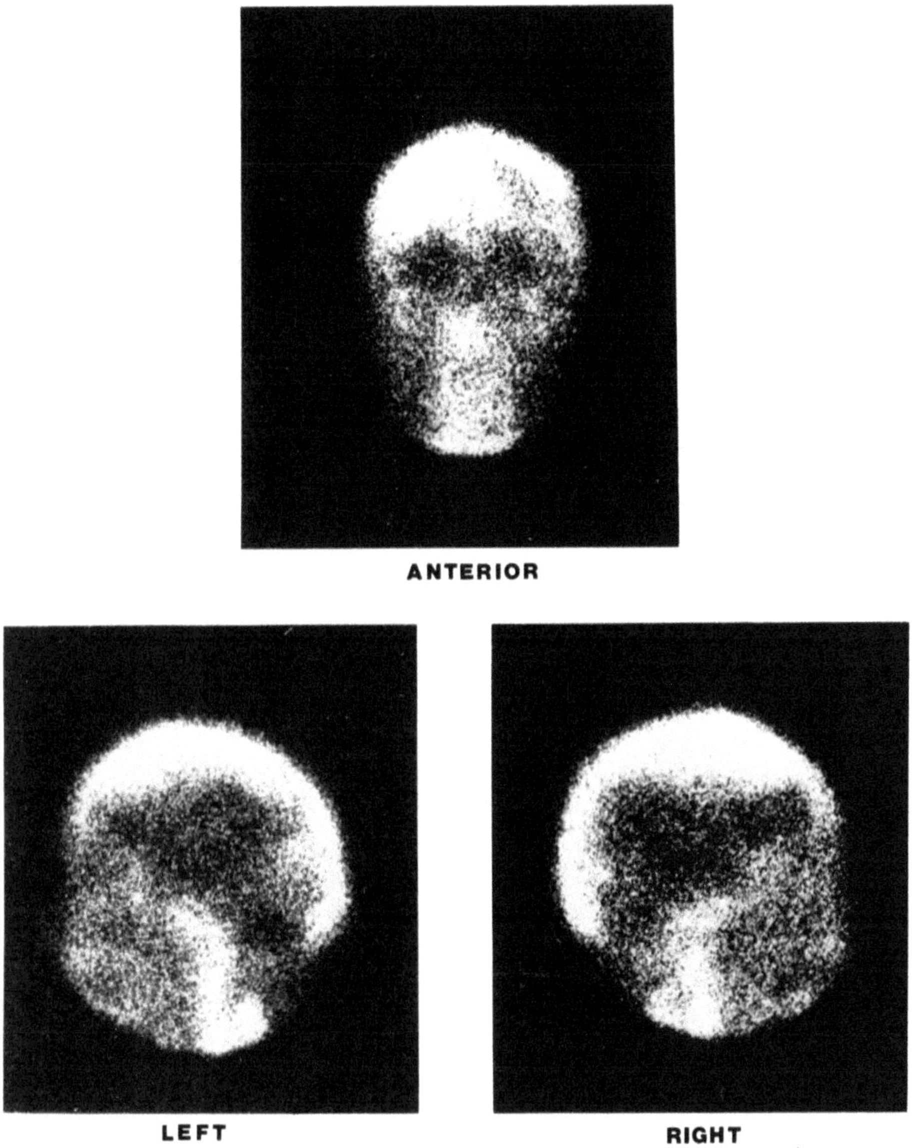

Fig. 5-6B. Camera images (anterior, left, and right lateral) show the skull lesions with a greater degree of resolution than the rectilinear views. Compare anterior camera with anterior rectilinear image.

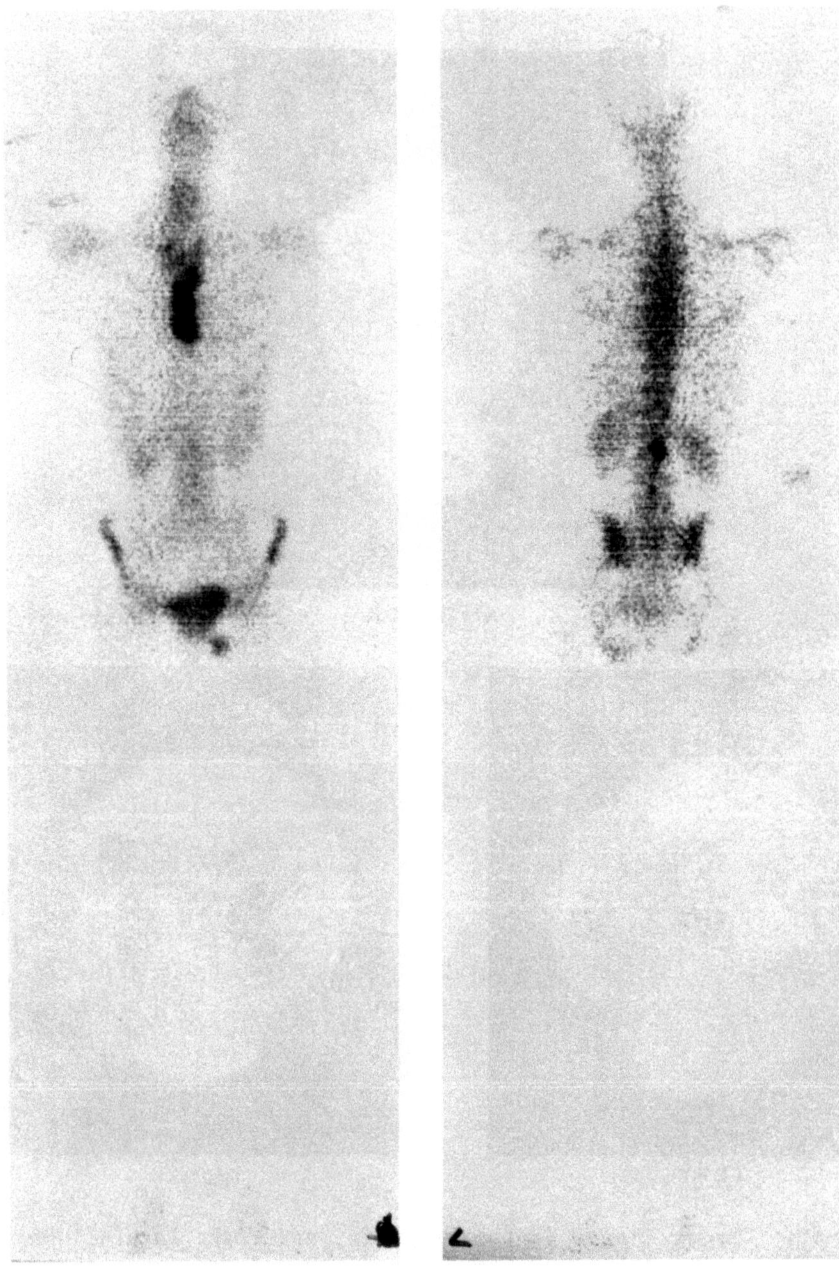

Fig. 5-7A. Initial anterior and posterior bone scan of this patient shows sternal uptake as well as an abnormal area of uptake in the lumbar spine. The focal activity noted beneath the bladder on the anterior view represents urine contamination.

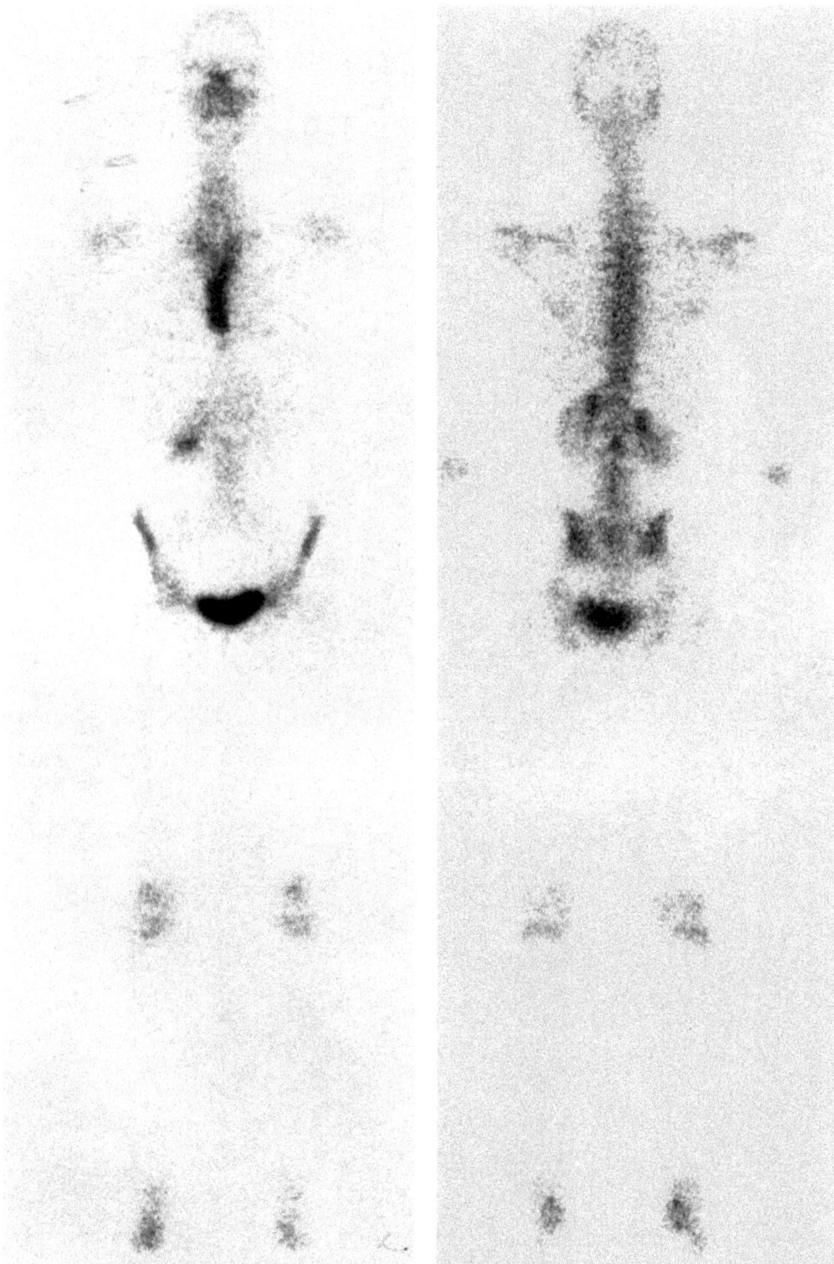

Fig. 5-7B. Follow-up study one year later, shows relatively less intense activity in the sternum and lumbar spine.

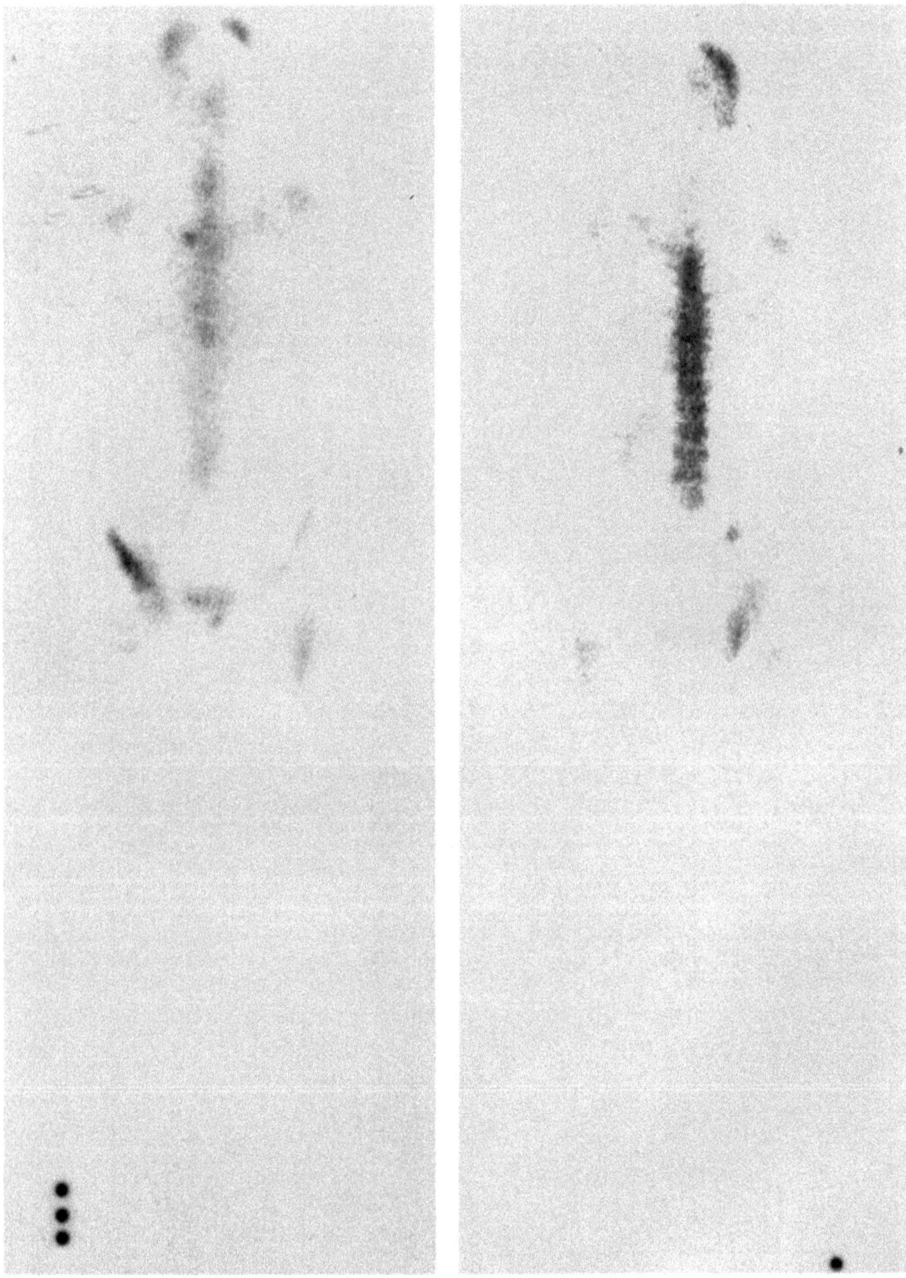

Fig. 5-8. Anterior and posterior bone scan of a patient with severe skeletal metastatic disease. Note less than normal uptake in the kidneys and no visualization of the soft tissues of the extremities. This may be partly due to preferential uptake by the large amount of skeletal tumor present.

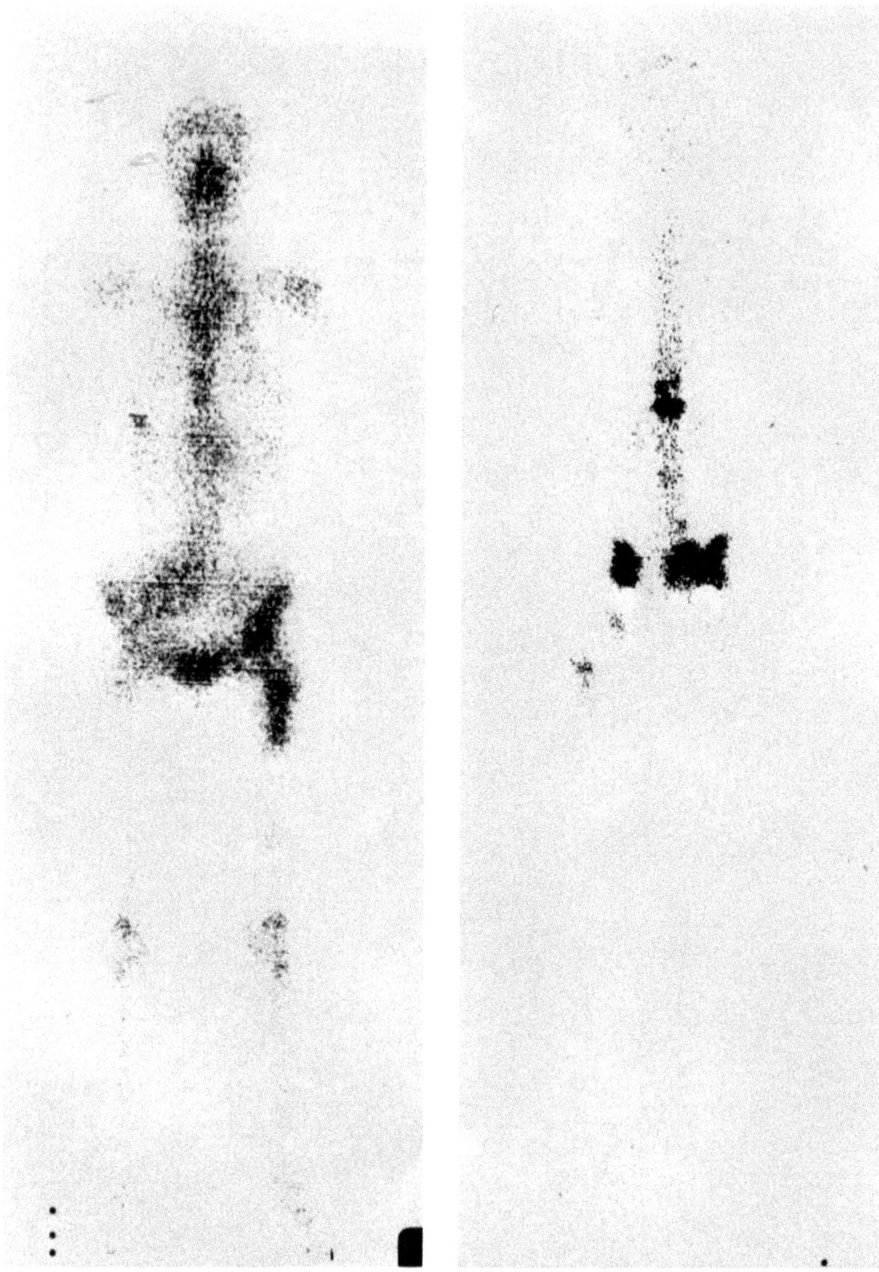

Fig. 5-9. Patient with extensive skeletal metastases. Anterior and posterior bone scan shows minimal soft tissue and renal localization.

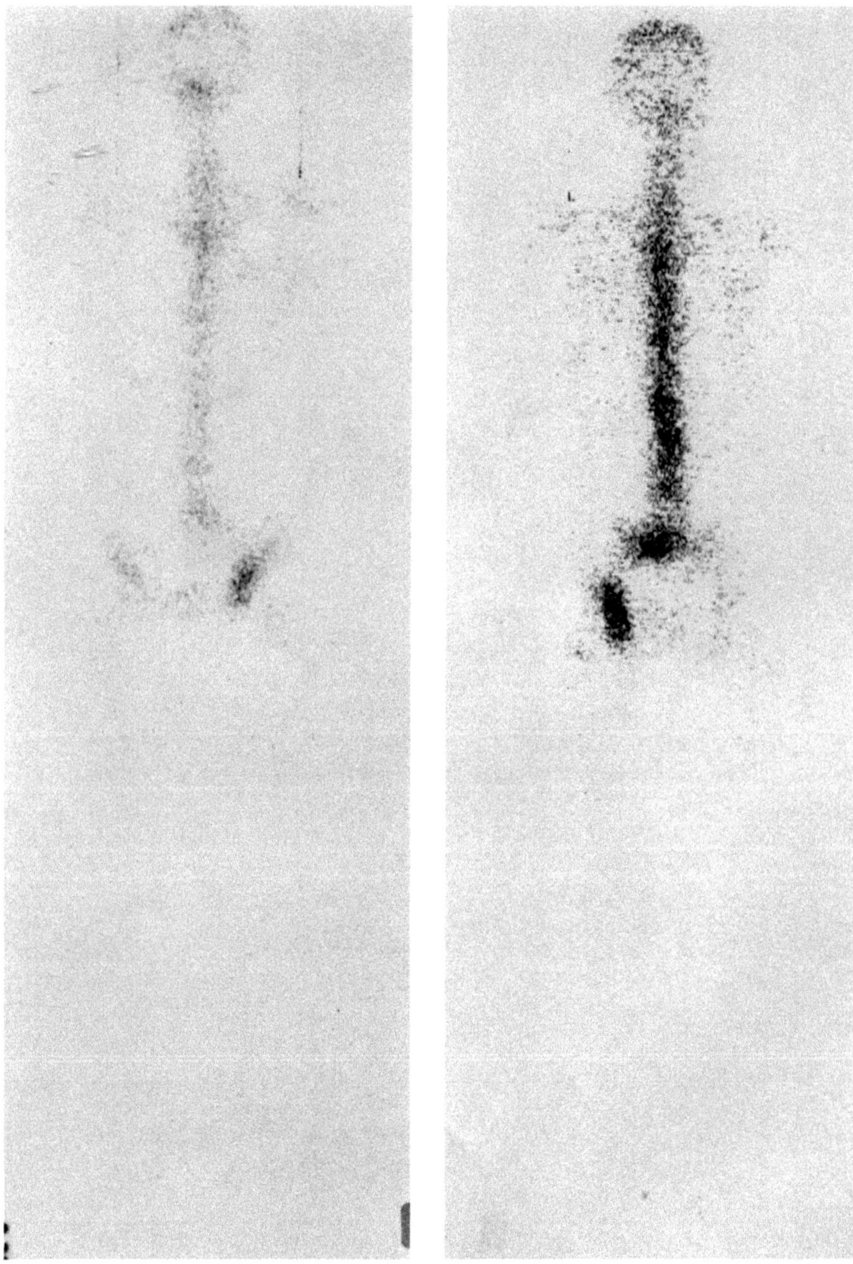

Fig. 5-10A. Anterior and posterior fluorine-18 skeletal scans reveal abnormal uptake in the sacrum and left ischium.

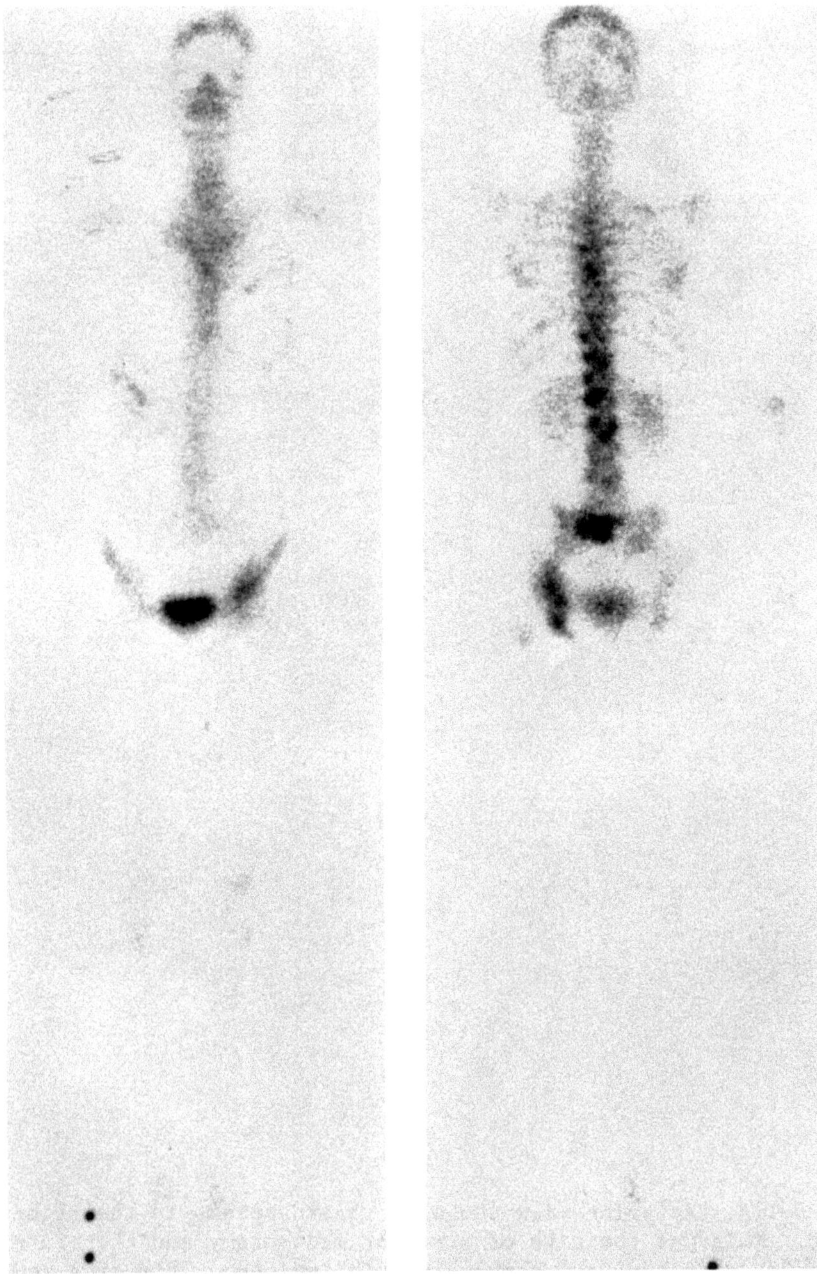

Fig. 5-10B. Study done with 99mTc polyphosphate within two months of the preceding fluorine-18 study shows far better detail and demonstrates several vertebral body lesions not visualized on the fluorine-18 scan.

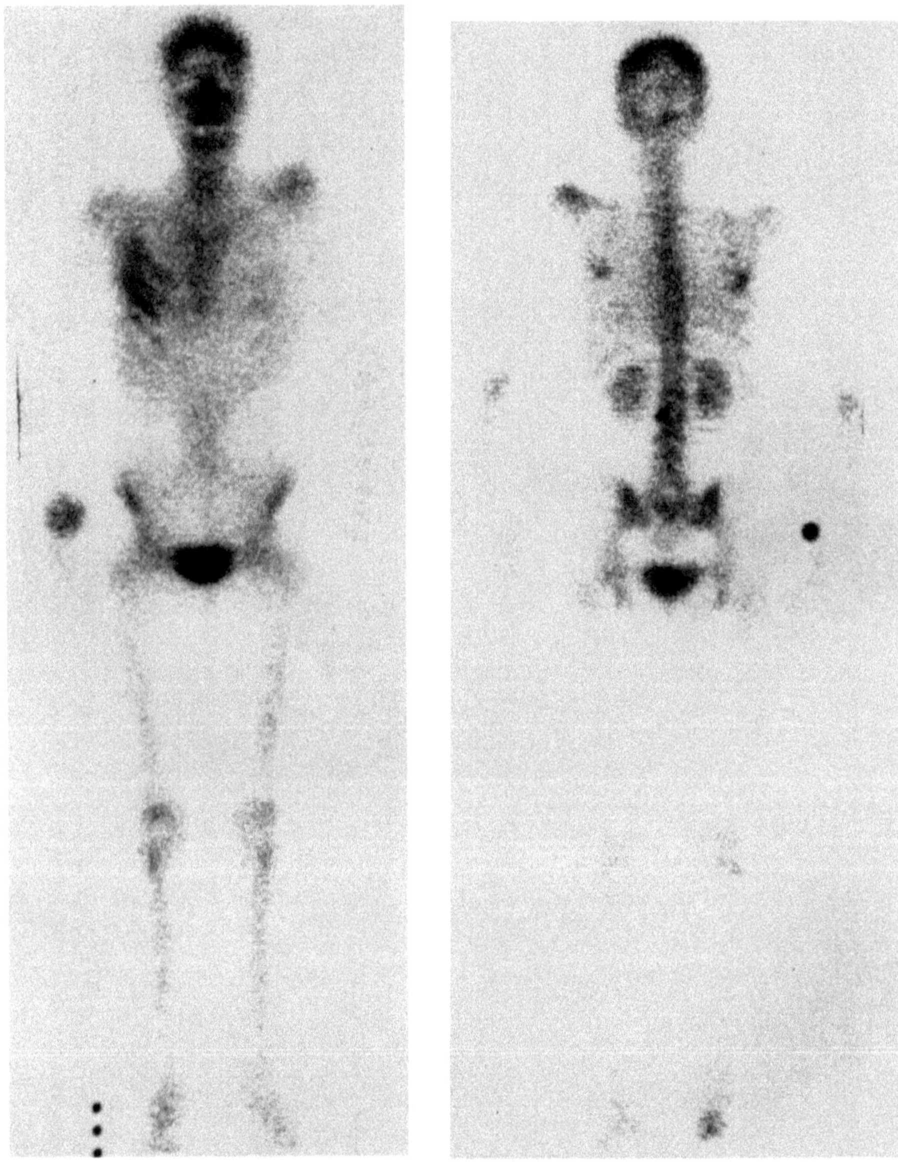

Fig. 5-11A. Anterior view shows increased uptake in the right upper chest. This was the site of a recent mastectomy and therefore could represent post-surgical changes or rib lesions. This area remained unchanged on several serial scans leaving the differential diagnosis unresolved. Rib radiographs were normal. Posterior view shows increased uptake in the region of L-2 vertebral body. Increased accumulation in the left shoulder was due to a chronic bursitis.

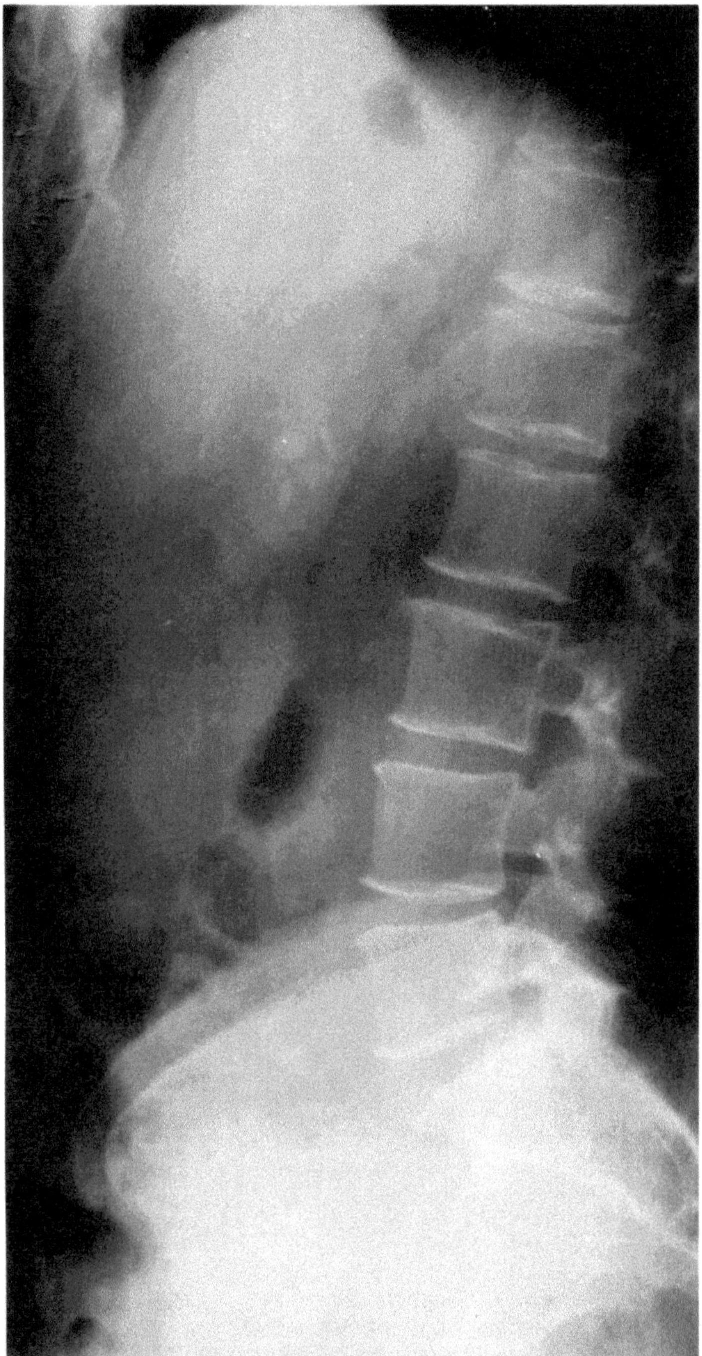

Fig. 5-11B. The radiograph of the spine was normal.

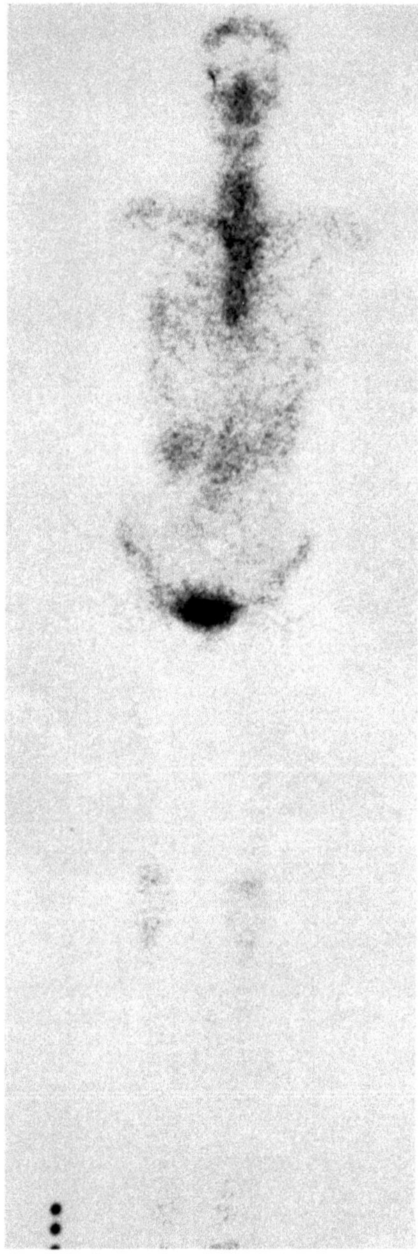

Fig. 5-12. This anterior scan shows slightly increased right chest wall uptake which was believed to be secondary to the patient's previous mastectomy. No areas of discrete increased uptake are seen, thus making rib lesions unlikely.

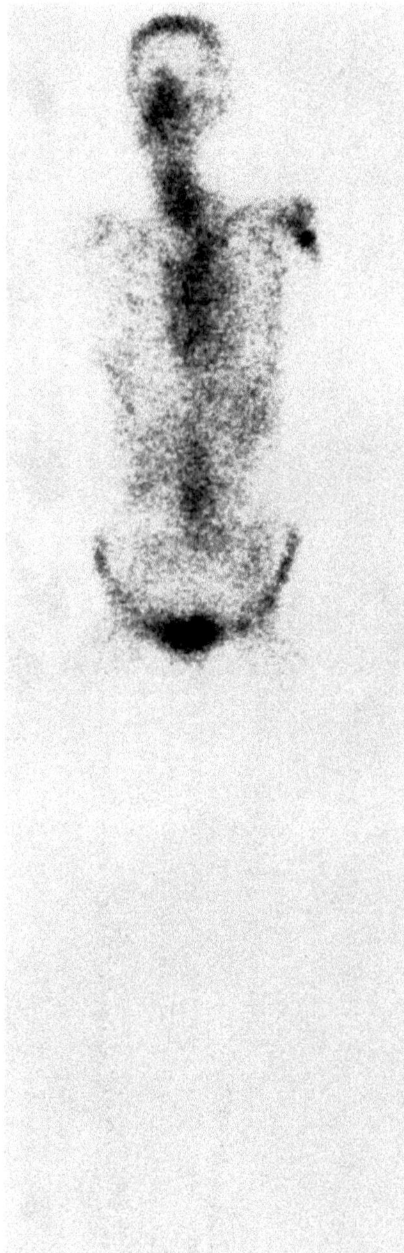

Fig. 5-13. Increased uptake in the left shoulder is secondary to recent trauma to the area. No metastases were identified on x-ray and the shoulder was normal on follow-up scan nine months later.

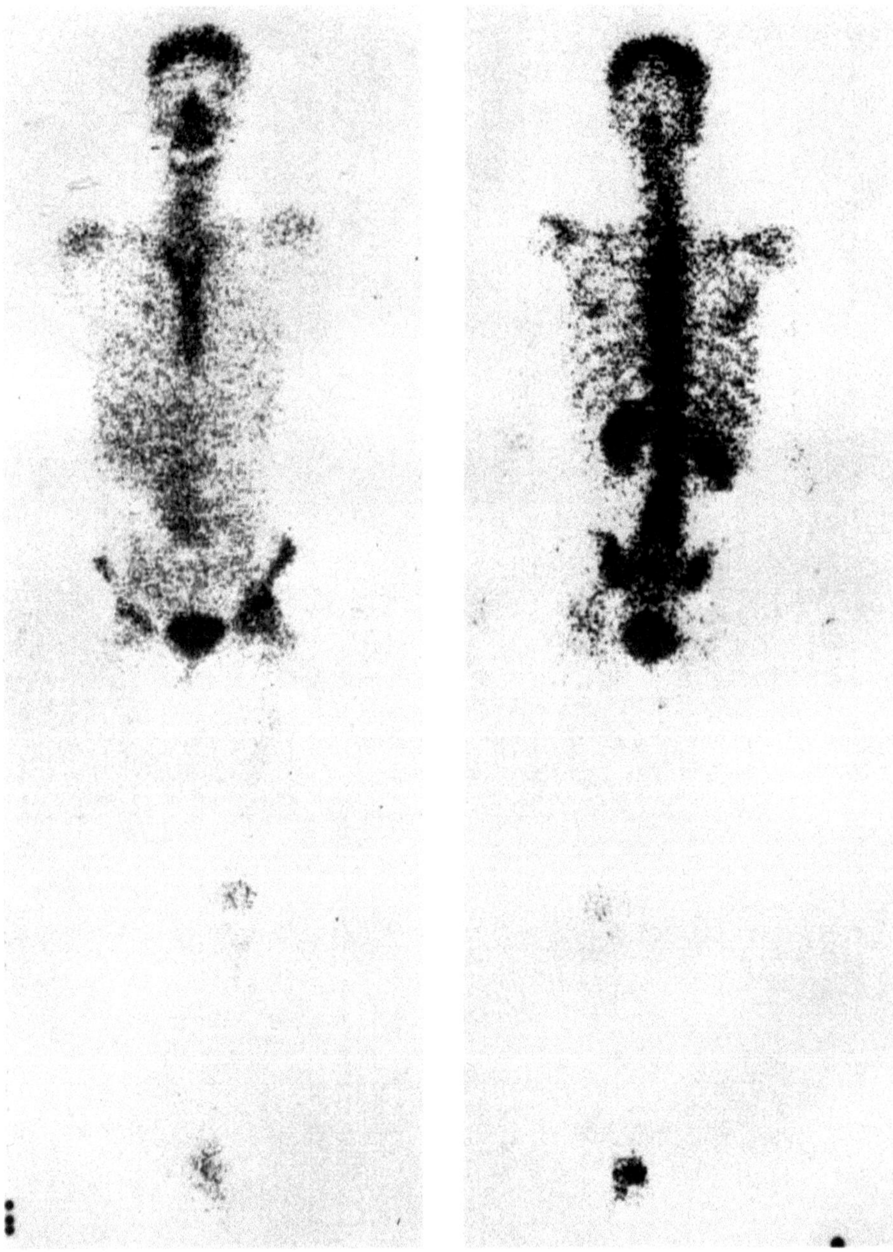

Fig. 5-14. Asymmetry of activity in the hip is present with less activity on the right side. This is due to poliomyelitis with right hemiatrophy. Left pelvic bone metastases, which might be suspected, were not present.

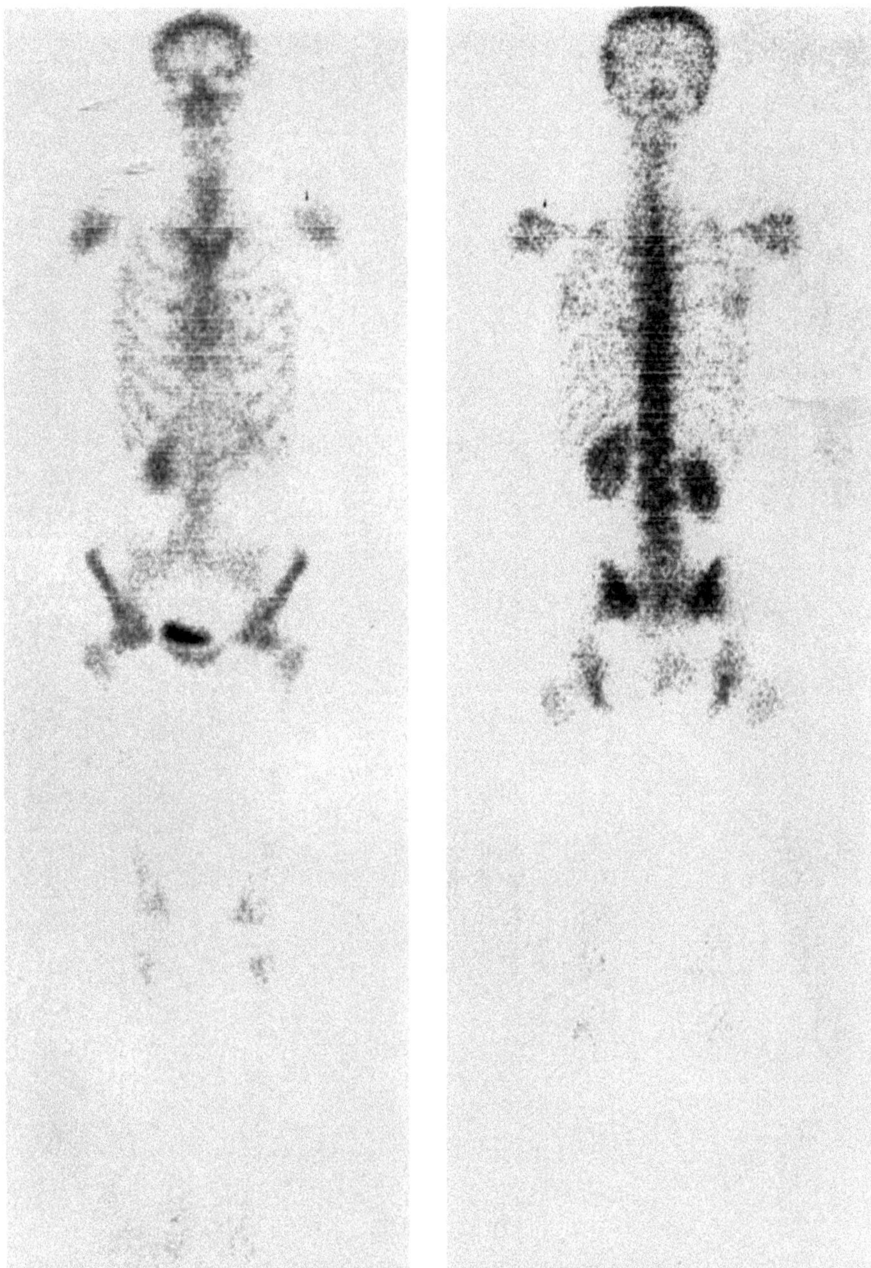

Fig. 5-15A. Anterior and posterior whole body bone scan showing uniform osseous localization of radionuclide with no skeletal asymmetry.

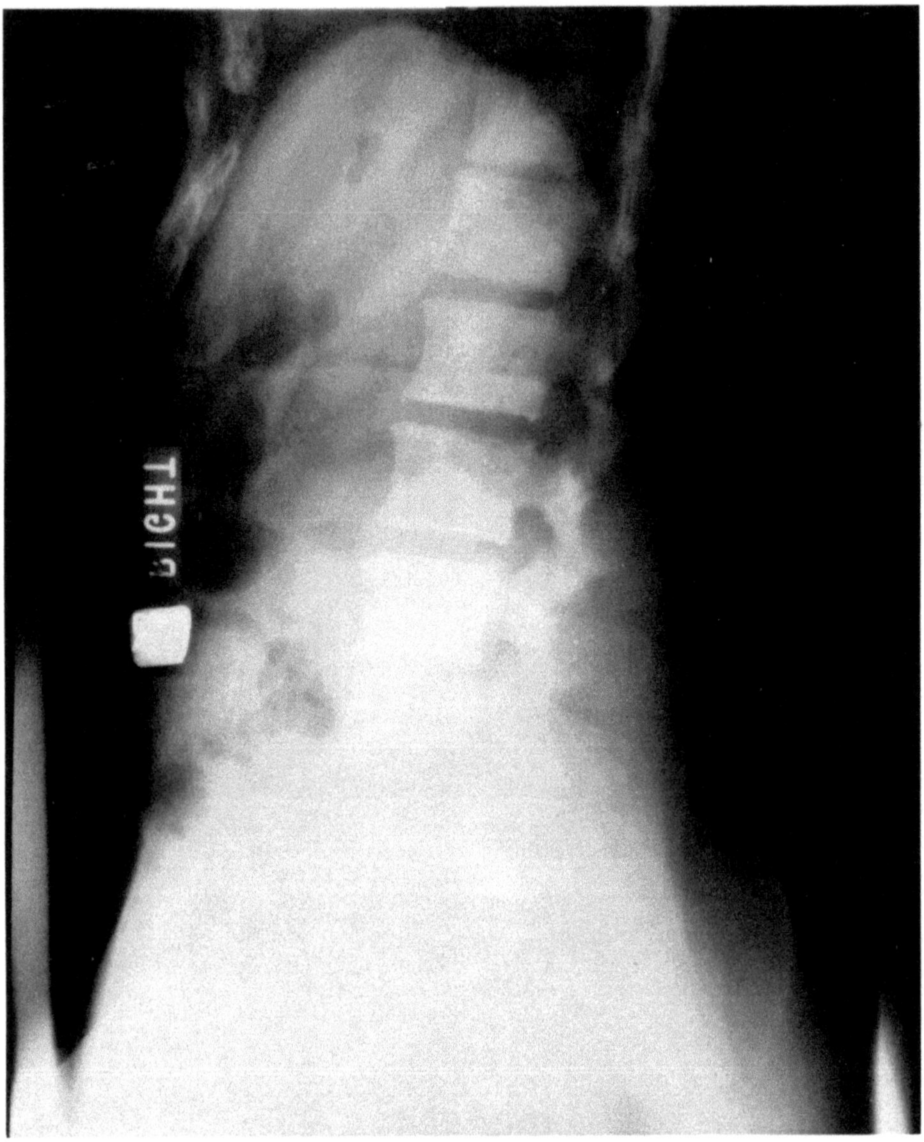

Fig. 5-15B

Fig. 5-15B,C,D. Metastases were found throughout the thoracic and lumbar spine, ribs, pelvis, and femurs.

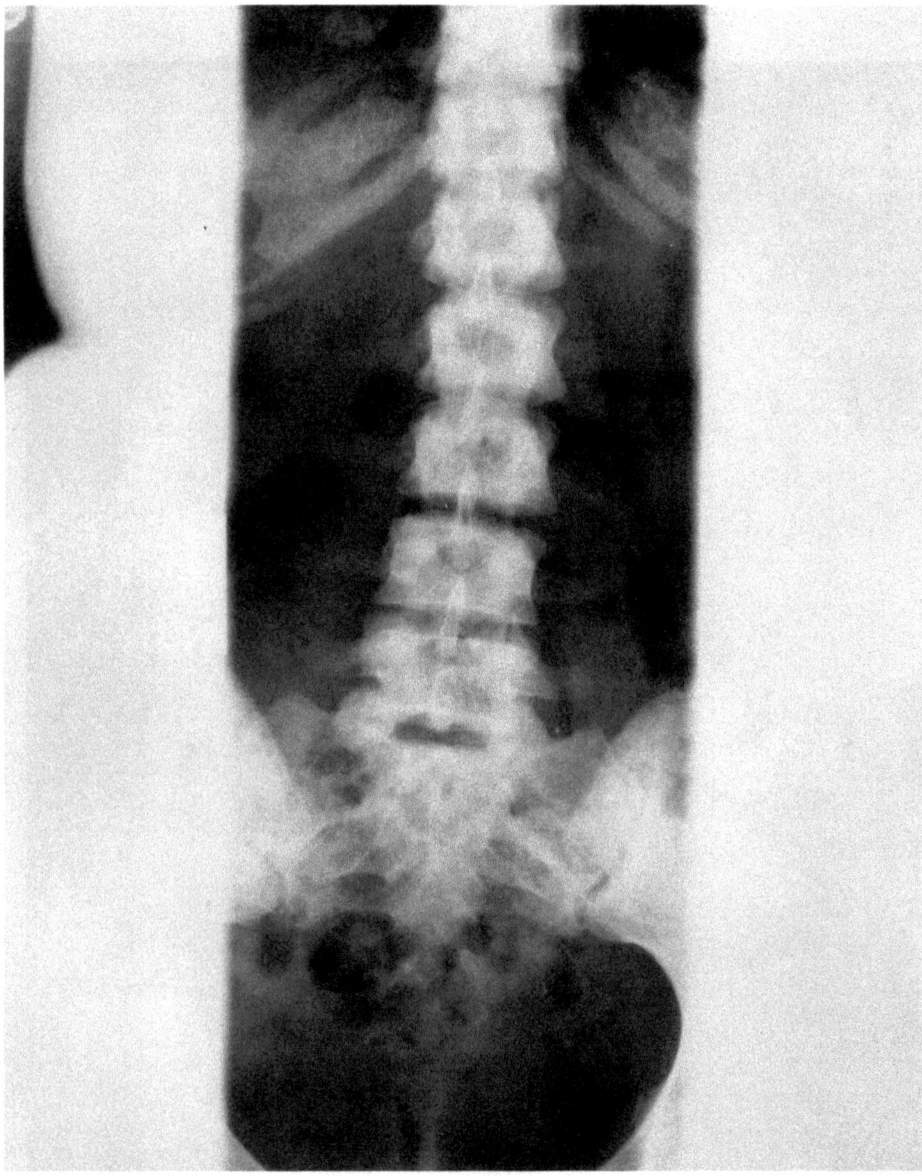

Fig. 5-15C

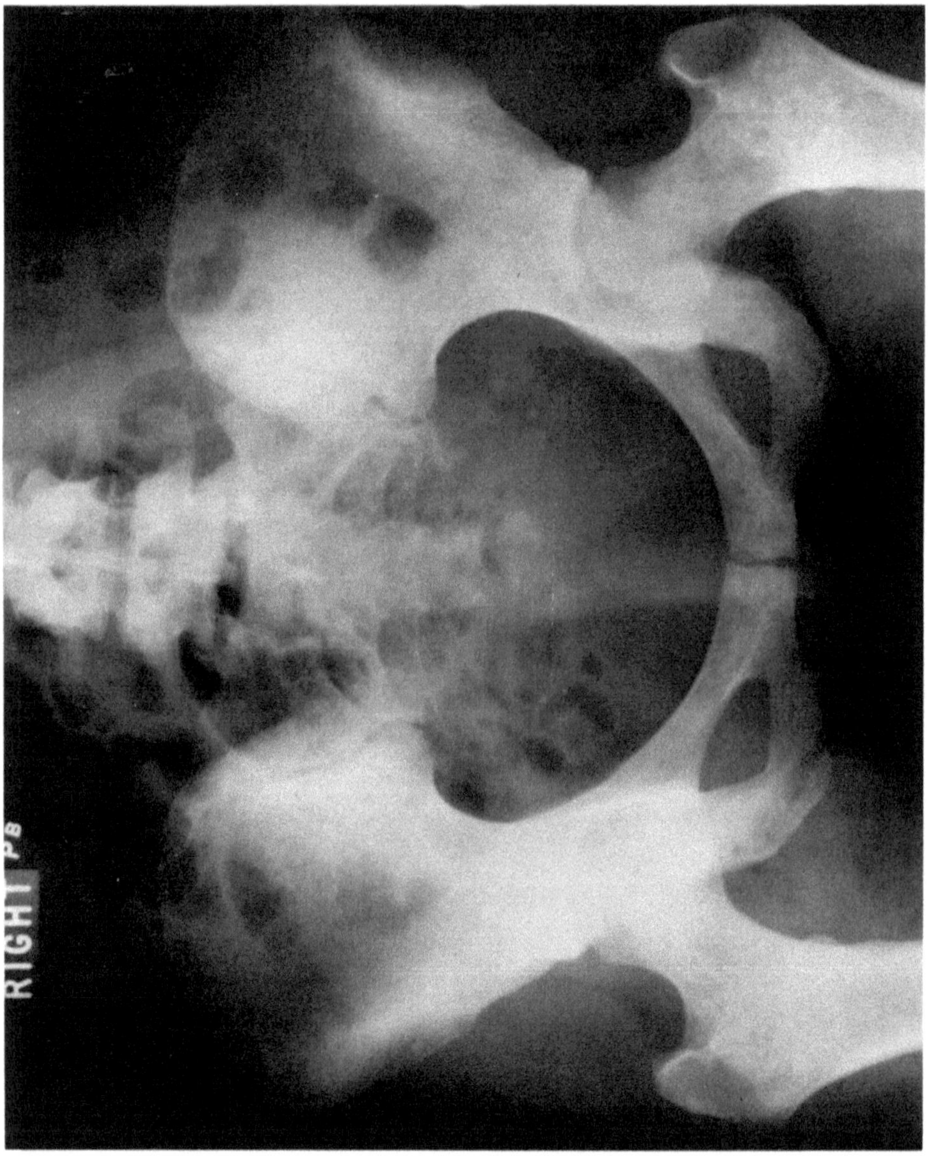

Fig. 5-15D

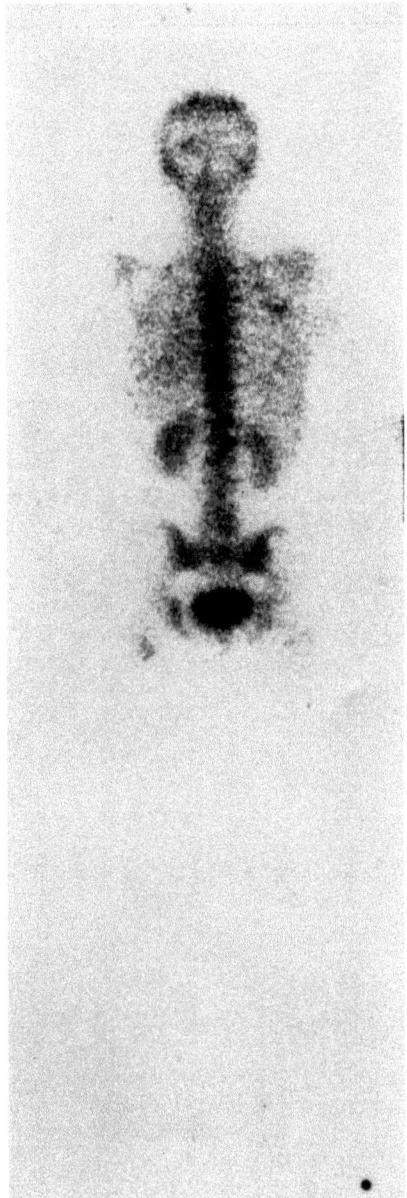

Fig. 5-16. Increased uptake in left femoral head is seen in this posterior bone scan. It corresponded in location to a bone island on the radiograph. The importance of correlating all scans with corresponding radiographs is obvious in order to avoid calling a benign bone lesion a metastasis.

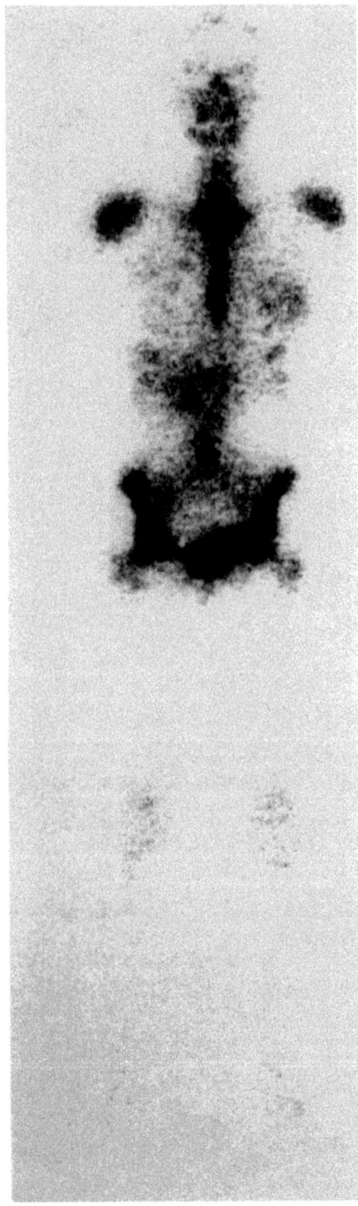

Fig. 5-17. This patient has a history of a right mastectomy one year prior to her present admission. The anterior 99mTc diphosphonate scan shows uptake of nuclide in the remaining left breast. Clinically and at surgery, the patient has a second carcinoma in this breast.

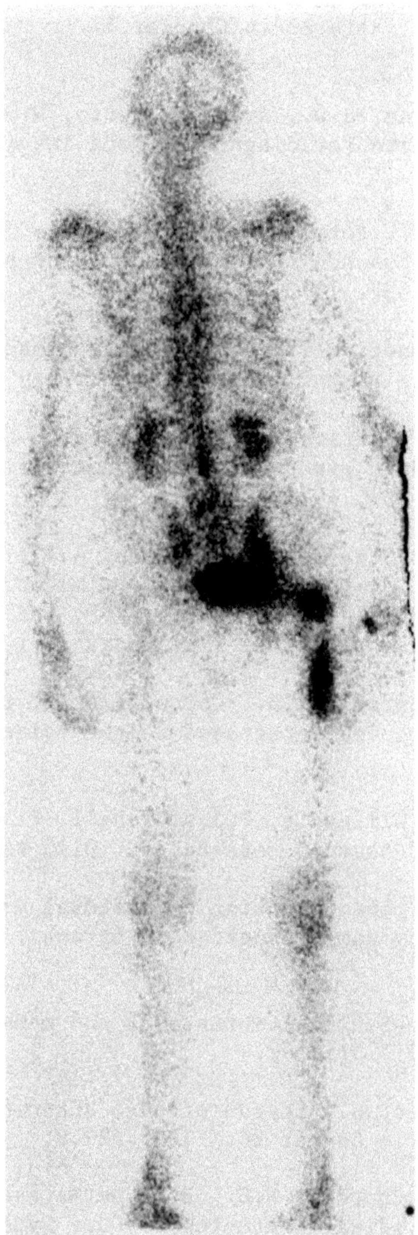

Fig. 5-18. A male patient with breast carcinoma. Posterior skeletal scintiscan shows increased uptake in the right femoral head and proximal femur. Originally interpreted as representing metastatic disease, this was proven to be Paget's disease by radiographic correlation.

References Chapter 5

1. Weber, D.A., Keyes, J.W., Jr., Benedetto, W.J., Wilson, G.A. Tc99m pyrophosphate for diagnostic bone imaging. Radiology 113: 131, 1974.

2. Penelegrass, H.P., Potsaid M.S., Castronovo, F.P. The clinical use of 99mTc diphosphonate: a new agent for skeletal imagery. Radiology 107: 557, 1973.

3. Hosain, P. Technetium-99m labelled pyrophosphate: a simple and reproducible bone scanning agent. Radiology 111: 255, 1974.

4. Fletcher, J.W., Solaric-George E., Henry, R.E., Donati, R.M. Evaluation of 99mTc pyrophosphate as a bone imaging agent. Radiology 109: 467, 1973.

5. Silberstein, E.B., Saenger, E.L. Tofe, A.J., Alexander, G.W., Jr., and Park, H.M. Imaging of bone metastases with 99mTc-Sn EHDP (diphosphonate), 18F, and skeletal radiography: a comparison of sensitivity. Radiology 107: 551, 1973.

6. Bachman, A.L., Sproul, E.E. Correlation of radiographic, autopsy findings in suspected metastases in the spine. Bull N Y Acad Med 31: 146, 1955.

7. Edelstyn, G.A., Gillespie, P.J., Greball, F. The radiological demonstration of osseous metastases. Clin Radiol 18: 158, 1967.

8. Galasko, C.S.B. The detection of skeletal metastases from mammary cancer by gamma camera scintigraphy. Brit J Surg 56: 757, 1969.

9. Galasko, C.S.B. Skeletal metastases and mammary cancer. Ann R Coll Surg Eng 50: 3, 1972.

10. Rubin, P., Ciccio, S. Status of bone scanning for bone metastases in breast cancer. Cancer 24: 1338, 1969.

11. Sklaroff, D.M., Charkes, N.D. Bone metastases from breast cancer at the time of radical mastectomy. Surg Gynec Obstet 127: 763, 1968.

12. Hoffman, H.C., Marty, R. Bone scanning: Its value in the preoperative evaluation of patients with suspicious breast Masses. Am J Surg 124: 194, 1972.

13. Hopkins, G.B., Kristensen, K.A.B. Whole body skeletal scintiphotography in the detection of occult breast carcinomas. Calif Med 119: 10, 1973.

14. Charkes, N.D., Young, I., Sklaroff, D.M. The pathologic basis of the strontium bone scan. JAMA 206: 2482, 1968.

15. Frankel, R.S., Richman, S.D., Levenson, S.M., Nelson, R.L., Ingle, J.N., Tormey, D.C., Jones, A.E., Johnston, G.S. Bone scintigraphy in breast carcinoma. J Nucl Med 15: 491, 1974.

16. Frankel, R.S., Jones, A.E., Cohen, J.A., Johnson, K.W., Johnston, G.S., Pomeroy, T.C. Clinical conditions of 67Ga and skeletal whole body radionuclide studies with radiography in Ewing's sarcoma. Radiology 110: 597, 1974.

17. Jones, A.E., Frankel, R.S., Di Chiro, G., Johnston, G.S. Brain scintigraphy with 99mTc pertechnetate, 99mTc polyphosphate, and 67Ga citrate. Radiology 112: 123, 1974.

18. Frankel, R.S., Johnson, K.W., Mabry, J.J., Johnston, G.S. "Normal" bone radionuclide image with diffuse skeletal lymphoma. A case report. Radiology 111: 365, 1974.

19. Thripkaew, A.K., Henkin, R.E., Quinn, J.L., III, False negative bone scans in disseminated metastatic disease. Radiology 113: 383, 1974.

20. Hattner, R.S., Miller, S.W., Schimmel, D. Significance of renal asymmetry in bone scans: Experience in 795 cases. J Nucl Med 16: 161, 1975.

21. Sharma, S.M., Quinn, J.L, III, Significance of 18 F-fluoride renal accumulation during bone imaging. J Nucl Med 13: 744, 1972.

CHAPTER 6

Gallium-67 Scintigraphy

Steven D. Richman, M.D.

Department of Nuclear Medicine
National Institutes of Health
Bethesda, Maryland

It has long been the ambition of nuclear medicine to provide a direct, tumor specific scanning agent, that has a specific affinity for neoplastic tissue. Thus far gallium-67 citrate (67Ga) is the tumor-seeking radionuclide which has achieved the greatest clinical success. Intensive investigations have demonstrated that a wide spectrum of neoplasms concentrate 67Ga to varying degrees (1,2)(Fig. 6-15).

Gallium-67, however, has proved a relatively insensitive agent for the detection of primary breast carcinoma. Higasi (3) studied 16 cases of breast carcinoma and eight were positive with 67Ga scintigraphy. Among nine patients with breast carcinoma, Langhammer (4) demonstrated only three with abnormal concentration of 67Ga. Lavender (5) was able to show increased 67Ga activity in two of ten primary malignancies. Five of seven patients had increased uptake in the series reported by Fogh (6). Our studies show a disappointing 52% detection rate for primary adenocarcinoma of the breast in 21 patients evaluated with 67Ga. Gallium-67 is not particularly suited to gamma camera scintigraphy and special breast views have not improved its diagnostic usefulness (see Chapter 4). Furthermore, several pitfalls in interpretation are encountered (Figs. 6-3,4). The complicating factor of physiologic 67Ga concentration in the prelactating and lactating breast is well documented (6,7). Women on cyclic hormones have demonstrated increased mammary uptake (8). Normal diffuse uptake might therefore mask a focal, pathologic accumulation. "False-positive" localization can occur, albeit infrequently, in fibrocystic breast disease (Figs. 6-3C,4B) and gynecomastia (3,9,10).

Gallium-67 is no substitute for roentgenographic examination of breast disease, and the search for an effective breast scanning agent continues. The role of 67Ga, however, need not be relegated to the preoperative evaluation of the primary tumor. We have studied 67Ga scintigraphy as a diagnostic adjunct in 104 patients either after mastectomy, or in inoperable cases, before therapy.

Whole body 67Ga scintigraphy was routinely performed 48-72 hours after intravenous administration of 35-50 uCi/kg body weight of 67Ga. A dual probe 5 inch crystal whole body scanner with 5:1 minification and a spectrometer window setting of 130-330KeV was used. Adequate bowel preparation to eliminate interfering 67Ga from the abdomen was necessary for accurate interpretation.

Eighty-three patients with evidence for metastatic breast carcinoma were studied. Gallium-67 proved less sensitive than skeletal scintigraphy for the detection of osseous metastases (Figs. 6-6,7,8,20). Corroboration of skeletal involvement occurred in 34 (65%) of 52 cases. In patients with multiple bony metastases, 67Ga often failed to concentrate in all sites of tumor. When both 67Ga and 99mTc diphosphonate were positive the bone lesions were better visualized with the latter agent (Fig. 6-8). In only two cases with known multiple metastases, did 67Ga identify an additional skeletal metastasis before either bone scintigraphy or roentgenogram examinations.

Gallium-67 failed to localize differentially in 20 of 25 cases with secondary hepatic neoplasm (Figs. 6-9,11,12). Twenty of these patients had focal defects on the 99mTc sulfur colloid liver scan. In two cases, metastatic tumor resulted in areas of preferential 67Ga localization corresponding with areas of diminished colloid uptake. Two patients had decreased 67Ga activity in the region of large liver scan defects. One patient with severe hepatic replacement had absent 67Ga uptake throughout the liver parenchyma (Fig. 6-11).

The accuracy of 67Ga for lung metastases was also disappointing; seven (35%) of 20 cases with roentgenographic evidence of pulmonary involvement had abnormal 67Ga uptake (Figs. 6-13,14).

With regard to individual organ tracer techniques, the 67Ga scan played a limited confirmatory role in the assessment of metastatic lesions. For serial follow-up of metastatic tumor, bone, brain, and liver scans consistently provided information far superior to the 67Ga scan. Occasionally 67Ga uptake provided an ancillary visual index of tumor involvement and was used in conjunction with isolated organ studies and roentgenographic examination.

In some patients with known metastatic tumor, 67Ga scintigraphy did demonstrate a unique diagnostic value. The detection of mediastinal involvement in eight cases (10%) of this select population was most rewarding (Figs. 6-5,6,16). Autopsy in two patients confirmed metastatic breast carcinoma. Mediastinoscopy, utilized to obtain tissue for hormone-receptor studies, was positive for metastatic breast carcinoma in four of five patients undergoing this procedure. In three biopsy-proven cases, 67Ga was the sole means of detection of mediastinal tumor in the presence of unremarkable chest roentgenograms and tomograms of the mediastinum.

Gallium-67 scintigraphy was performed in 21 post-surgical patients in whom all other parameters indicated a disease-free status. Gallium-67 scanning provided a useful, objective procedure corroborating the absence of metastases in 20 cases. Although 67Ga scans were negative in 20 of the patients, in one instance 67Ga demonstrated occult mediastinal tumor as the only evidence for metastasis. Therapy was instituted and the follow-up 67Ga scan returned to normal.

Gallium-67 scanning is a limited corroborative modality in both primary and metastatic breast carcinoma. Gallium-67 scanning cannot replace organ-specific radionuclide studies nor available clinical, laboratory and roentgenographic indices of tumor involvement. However, 67Ga has been most valuable for the detection of mediastinal breast metastases. Since documentation of the total extent and activity of metastatic disease is important for prognosis and therapy, the 67Ga scan scan can contribute useful information especially in breast carcinoma patients with known metastatic disease. Judicious use of 67Ga scintigraphy is recommended in the preoperative patient and as a screening procedure in postoperative patients without other evidence for metastases.

Finally, the propensity of 67Ga to concentrate in inflammatory lesions can be of considerable clinical value (11,12) since 67Ga has been used successfully to localize and follow inflammatory processes in the septic patient (Fig. 6-20) with breast carcinoma.

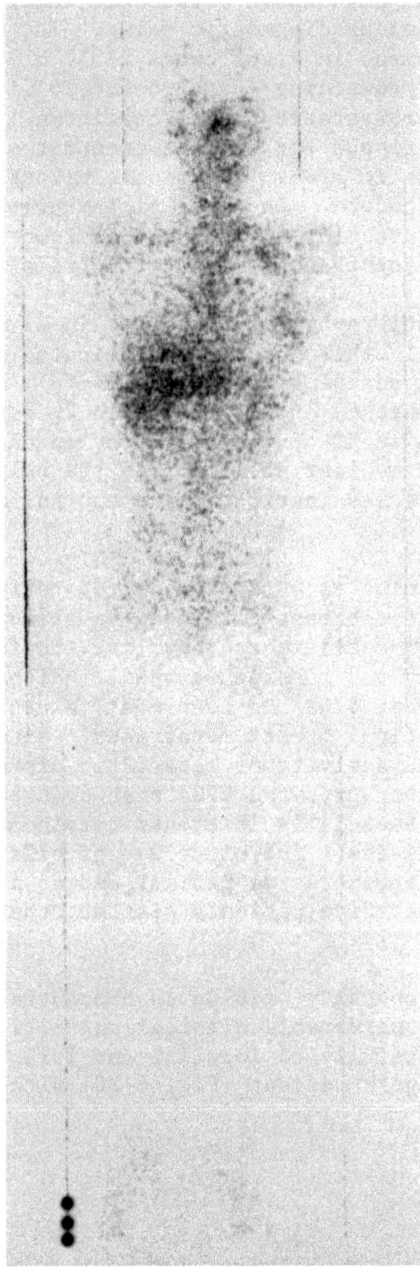

Fig. 6-1. Anterior whole body 67Ga scan of a 51 year-old woman with carcinoma of the left breast. The scan shows increased 67Ga uptake in the primary tumor. There is also increased activity in the left axillary region. Radical mastectomy was performed and 25 of 26 nodes were positive for metastases.

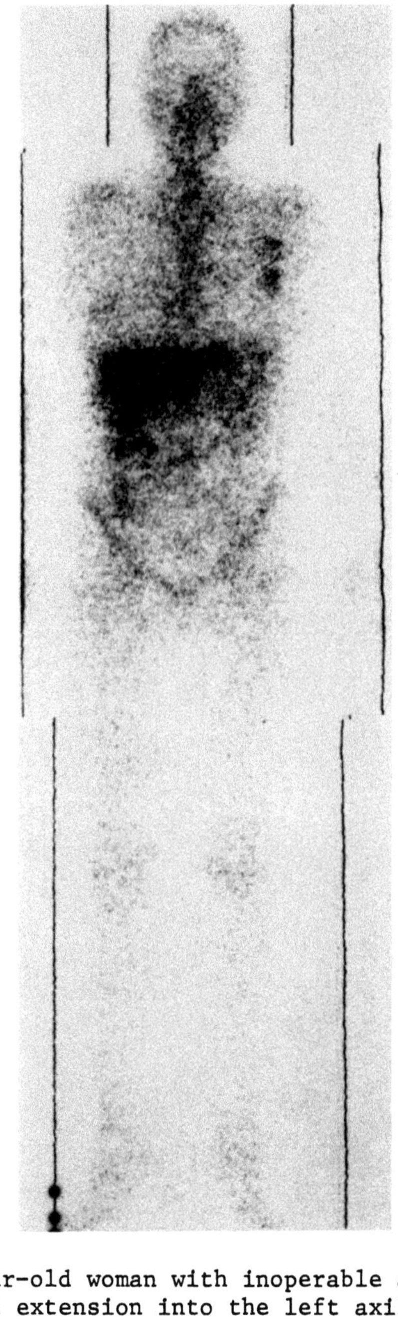

Fig. 6-2. A 62 year-old woman with inoperable adenocarcinoma of the left breast and extension into the left axilla. Increased 67Ga activity is shown in the primary tumor, the left axilla and the right breast. Mammography demonstrated only fibrocystic disease in the right breast, but clinical examination confirmed metastatic involvement.

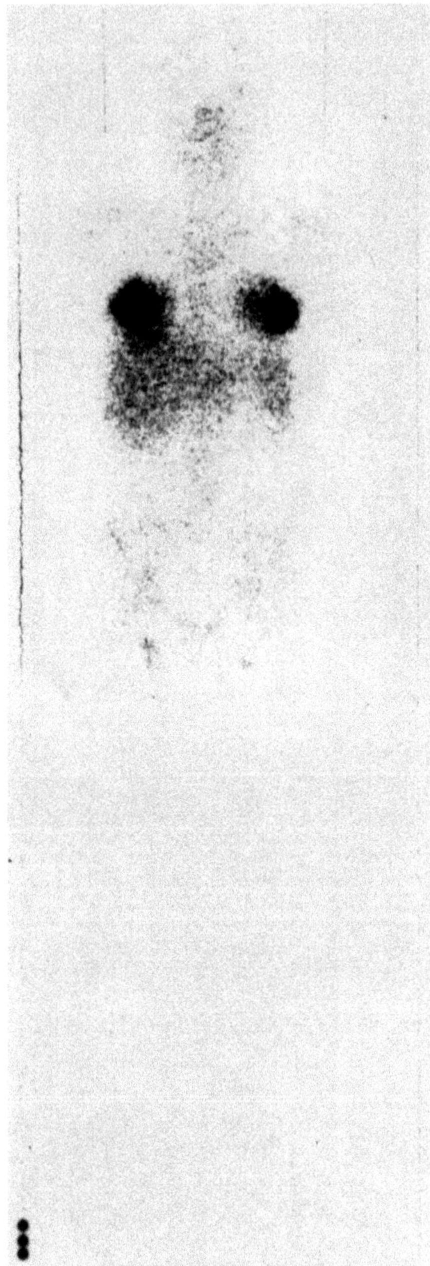

Fig. 6-3A. Pitfalls in interpretation, diffuse breast activity: Intense 67Ga activity, in a post-partum lactating patient with lymphoma. Note abnormal inguinal nodes.

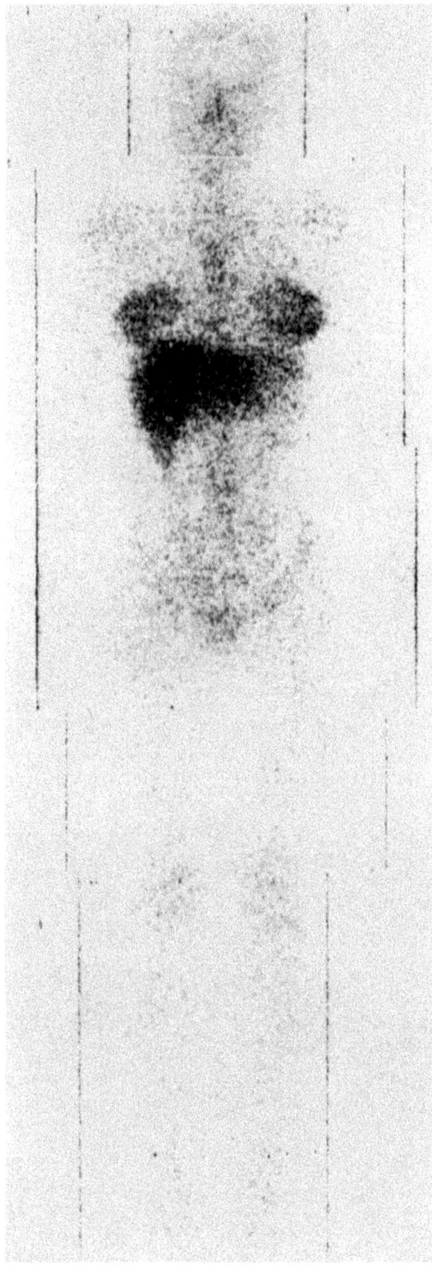

Fig. 6-3B. Pitfalls in interpretation, diffuse breast activity: Physiologic breast activity in a 21 year-old woman taking birth control pills. There was no evidence for breast disease.

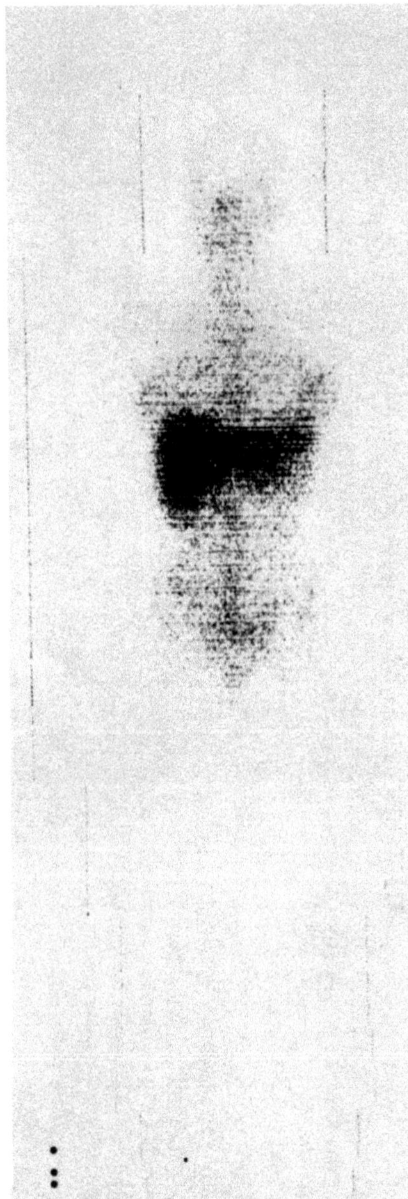

Fig. 6-3C. Pitfalls in interpretation, diffuse breast activity: Diffuse mammary uptake in a 39 year-old patient with fibrocystic disease of the right breast and a fibroadenoma in the left breast.

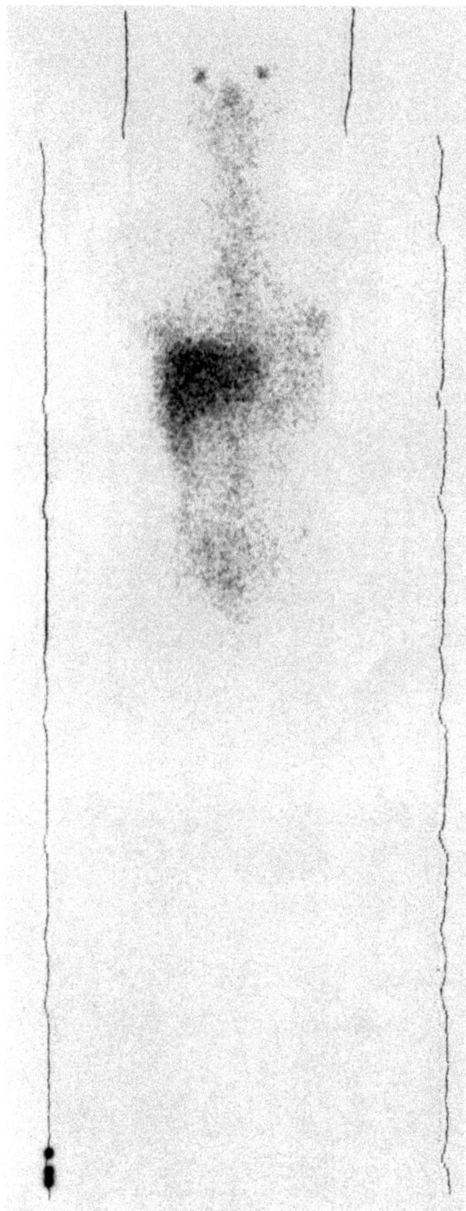

Fig. 6-3D. Adenocarcinoma of the right breast in a 41 year-old woman. Mammography indicated a malignancy. Bilateral, diffuse breast uptake would obscure any focal 67Ga abnormality.

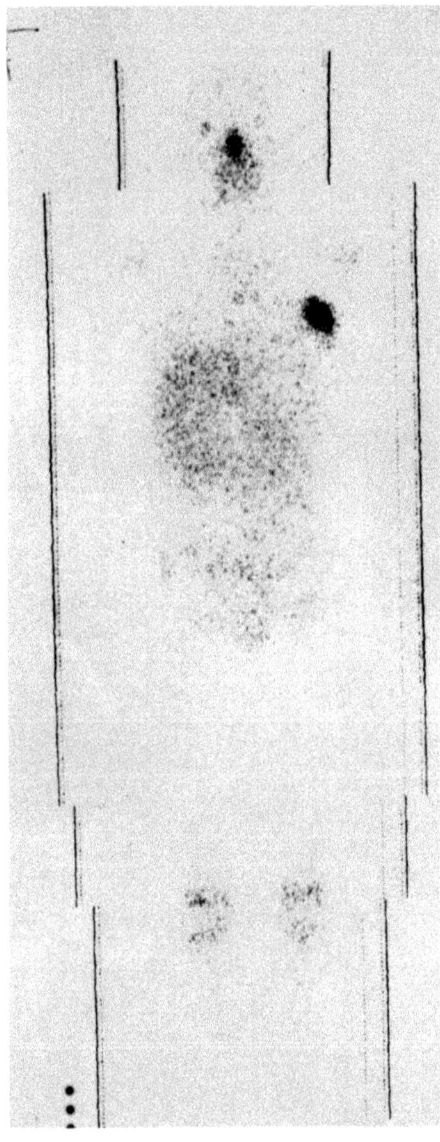

Fig. 6-4A. Pitfalls, focal abnormality: Discrete activity in left breast of a 15 year-old girl with acute myeloblastic leukemia. Biopsy revealed a myeloblastoma. (Intense nasopharyngeal 67Ga activity represents an abnormal mass as well).

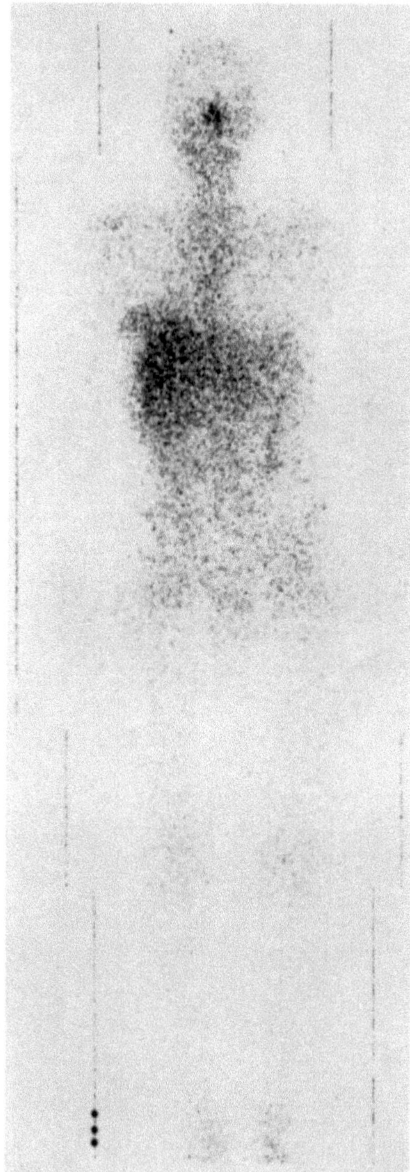

Fig. 6-4B. Pitfalls, focal abnormality: Focal activity representing fibrocystic disease in the right breast of a 50 year-old woman. Left radical mastectomy was performed one year prior to the 67Ga scan. Clinical examination of the right breast was normal and mammography showed only minimal fibrocystic change.

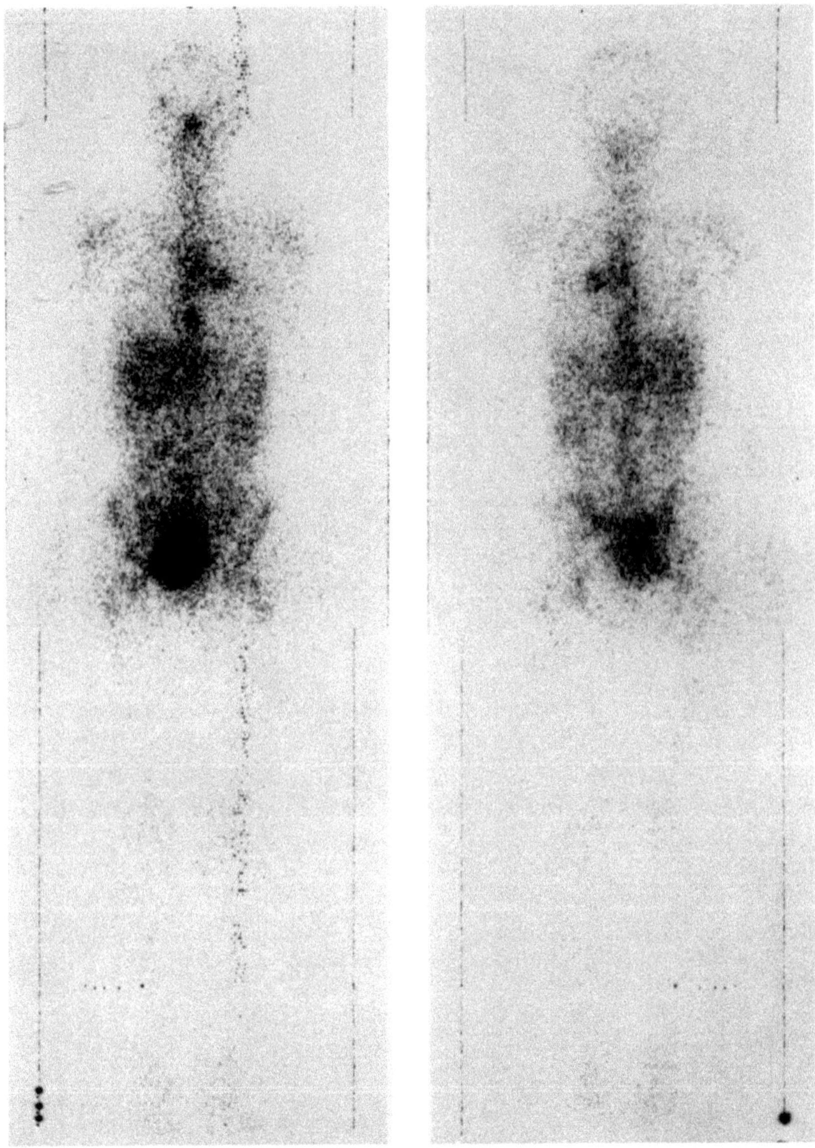

Fig. 6-5. The patient is a 31 year-old woman with bilateral mastectomies. Bone scan and roentgenographic examination of the sternum demonstrated lytic metastases. Anterior and posterior 67Ga views showed sternal metastases and also demonstrated abnormal uptake in the left hilum. Chest roentgenograms and tomography were unremarkable. Mediastinoscopy was positive for metastatic breast carcinoma. (Artifact is seen in the left leg and external to the skull).

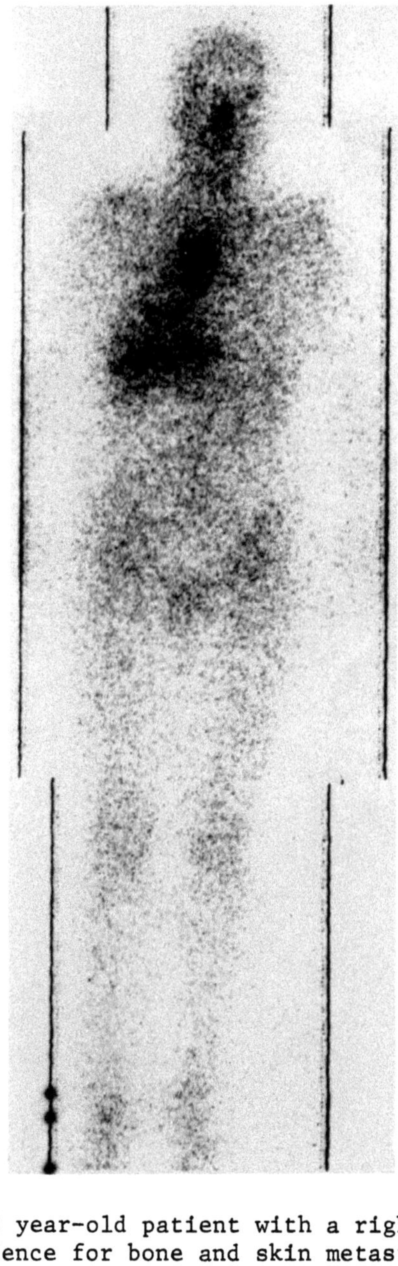

Fig. 6-6A. This 62 year-old patient with a right radical mastectomy and evidence for bone and skin metastases also has metastatic disease in the mediastinum. Gallium-67 failed to localize in the known metastases, but revealed mediastinal tumor in this previously unsuspected site of involvement.

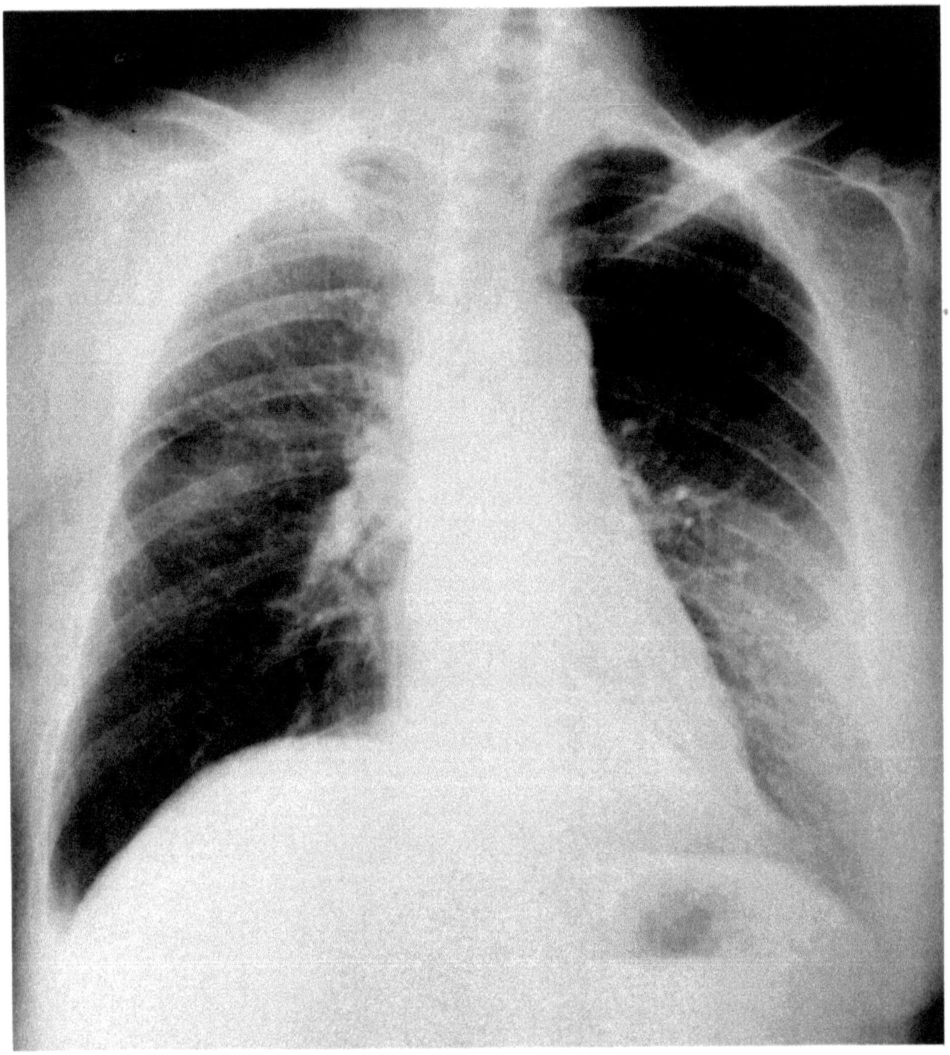

Fig. 6-6B. Chest roentgenogram and tomography failed to disclose the mediastinal tumors.

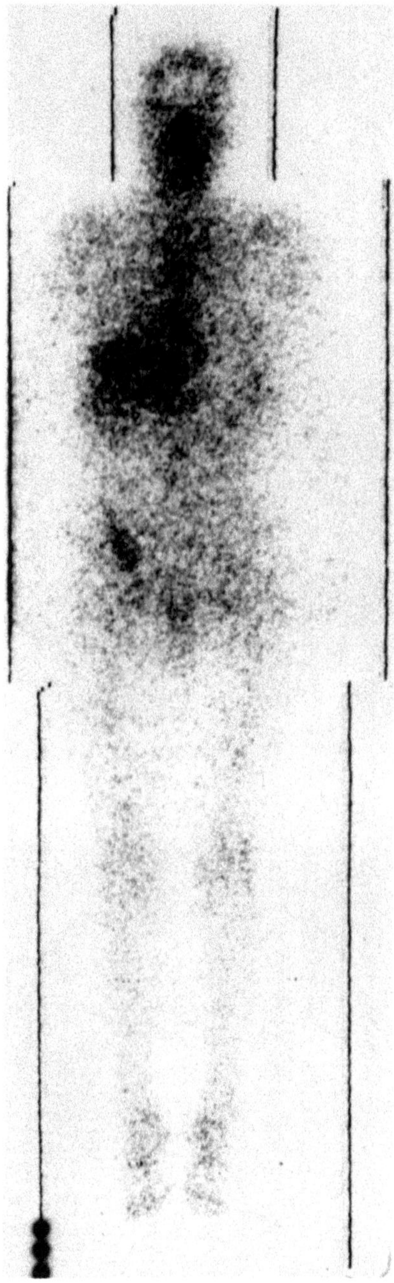

Fig. 6-6C. Following combination chemotherapy the 67Ga scan reverted to normal.

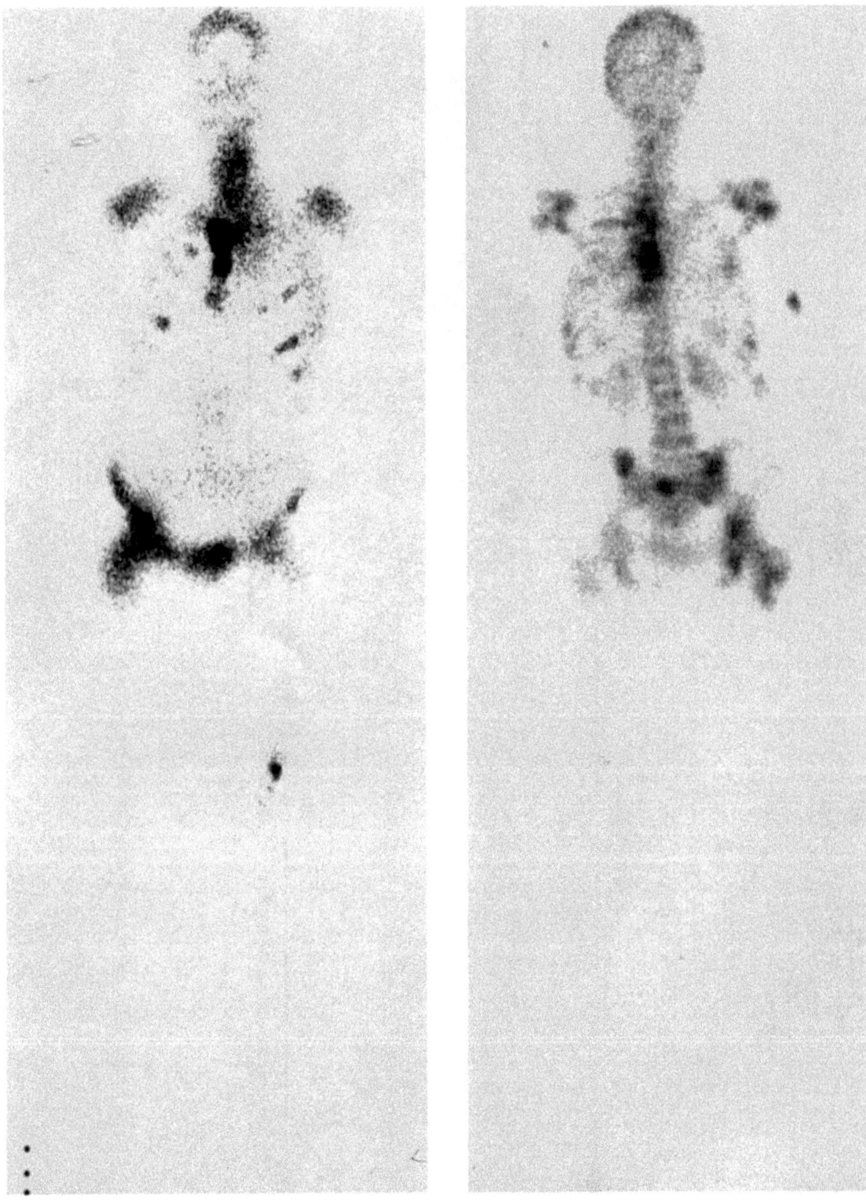

Fig. 6-7A. Anterior and posterior 99mTc diphosphonate bone scan demonstrates multiple sites of metastatic breast carcinoma.

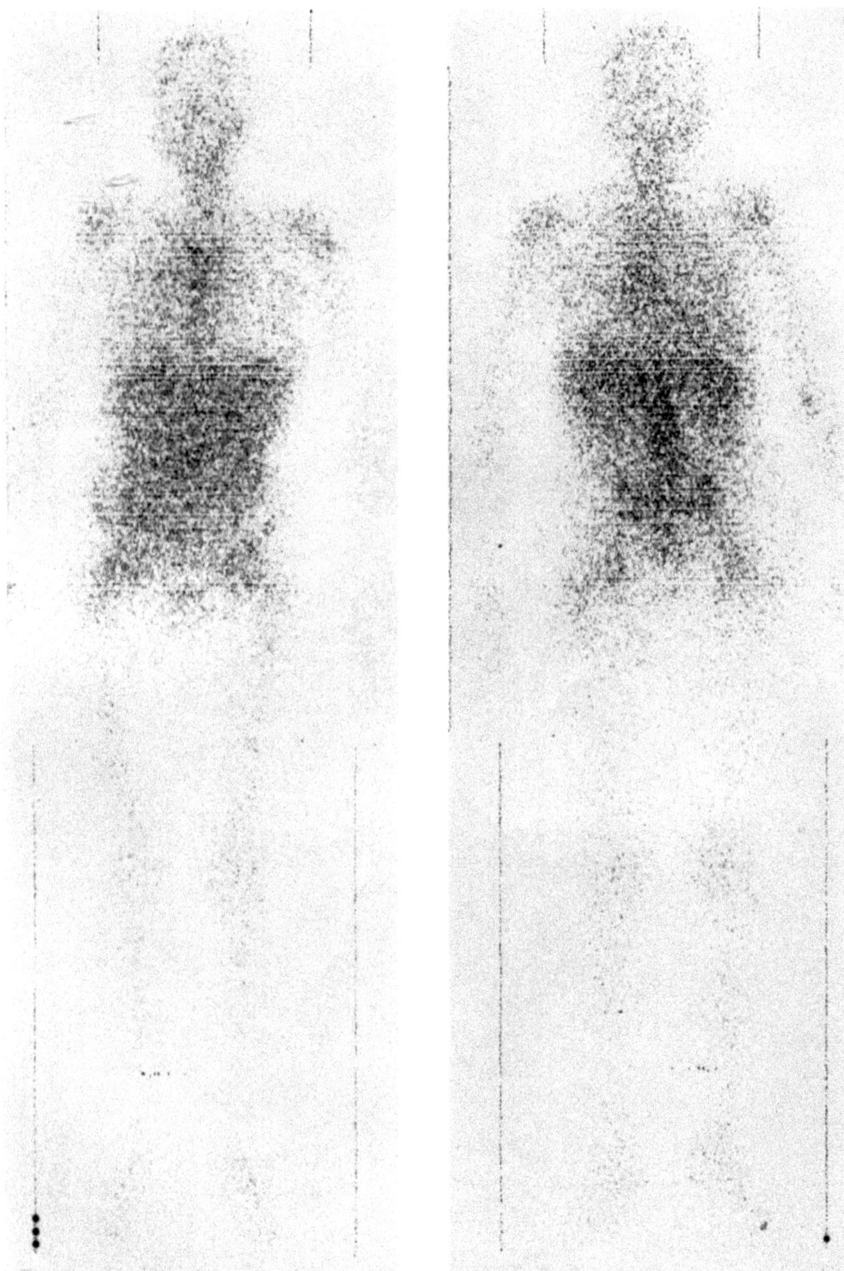

Fig. 6-7B. Anterior and posterior 67Ga scan failed to identify any bony metastases.

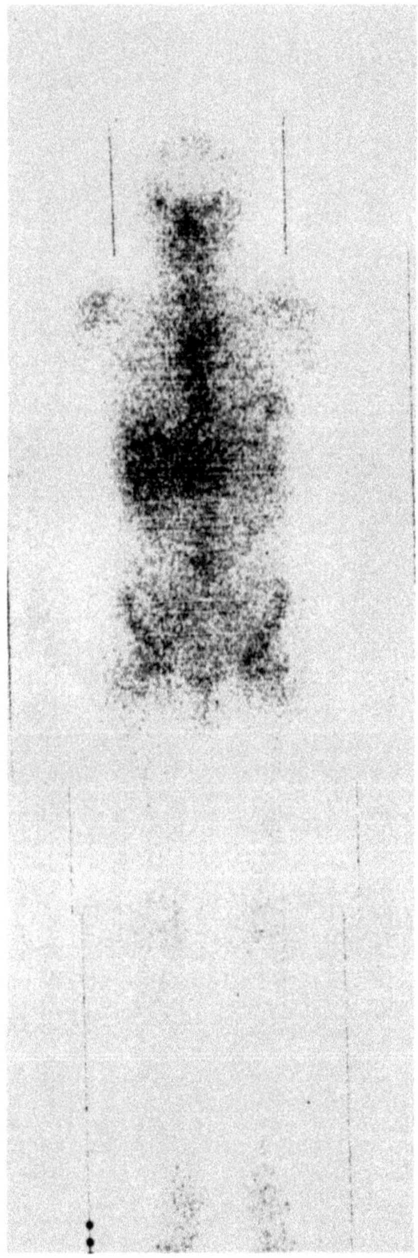

Fig. 6-8A. Anterior 67Ga shows questionable faint abnormal tracer in the sternum and left lower rib cage.

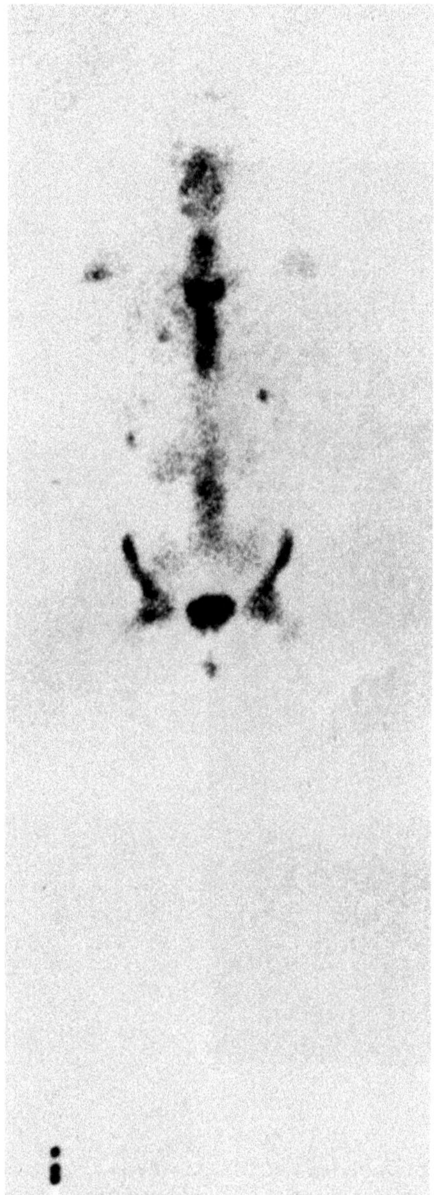

Fig. 6-8B. The bone scan with 99mTc diphosphonate reveals more intense uptake in the corresponding regions and demonstrates additional metastases in the right shoulder, right rib cage and in the right hip.

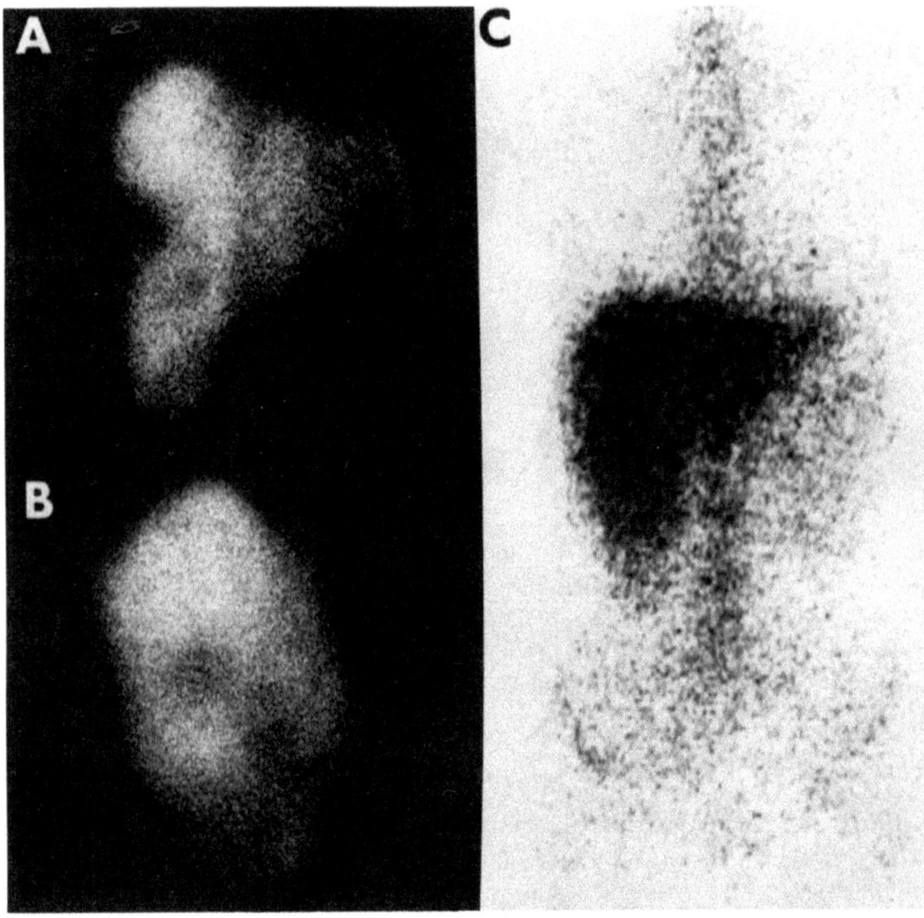

Fig. 6-9. Biopsy proven metastatic breast carcinoma involving the liver of a 31 year-old woman. Scintigraphy reveals hepatomegaly and large focal defects A) anterior, B) right lateral. Gallium-67 scan shows enlargement but no hepatic metastases are apparent (C).

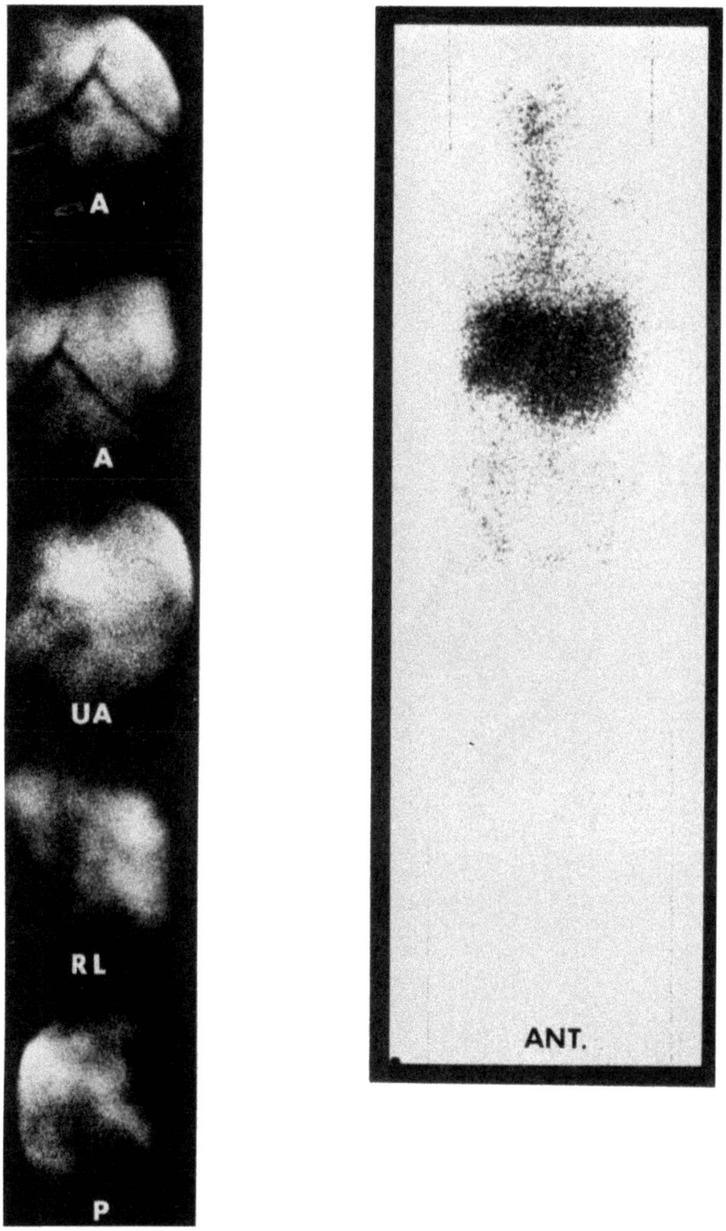

Fig. 6-10. There is increased 67Ga activity seen on the anterior whole body view in the right lobe of the liver which corresponds with the region of decreased liver activity on the 99mTc sulfur colloid views. Secondary hepatic neoplasm accounted for parenchymal replacement (Gamma camera images from top: A = reclining view with rib markers; A = reclining view including left hepatic lobe with rib markers; UA = upright anterior; RL = upright right lateral; P = upright posterior).

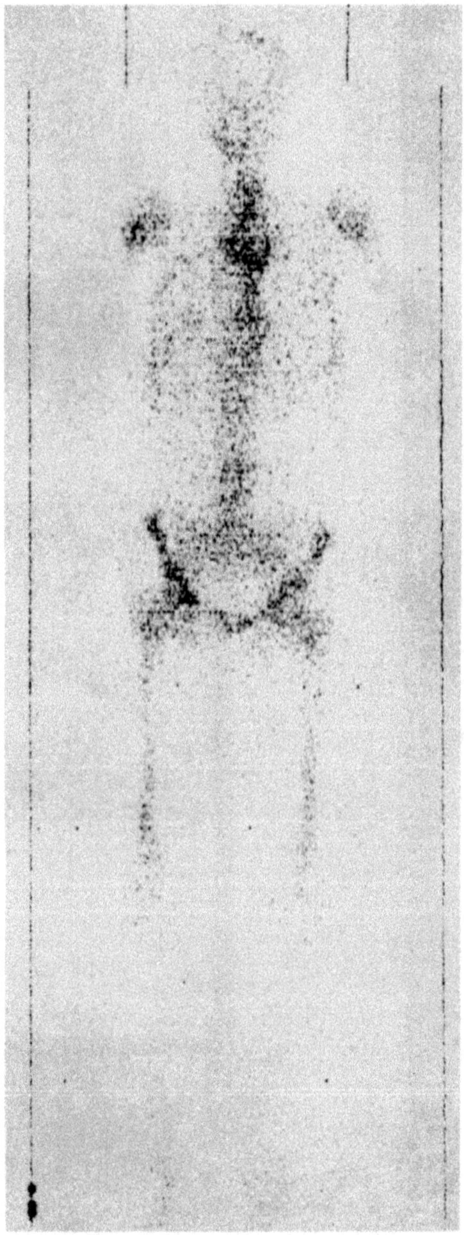

Fig. 6-11. Anterior whole body 67Ga scan of a 37 year-old patient with a previous right mastectomy and severe liver replacement by metastases. There is no 67Ga uptake by the liver. Well defined bony concentration, in part, reflects widely disseminated osseous metastases.

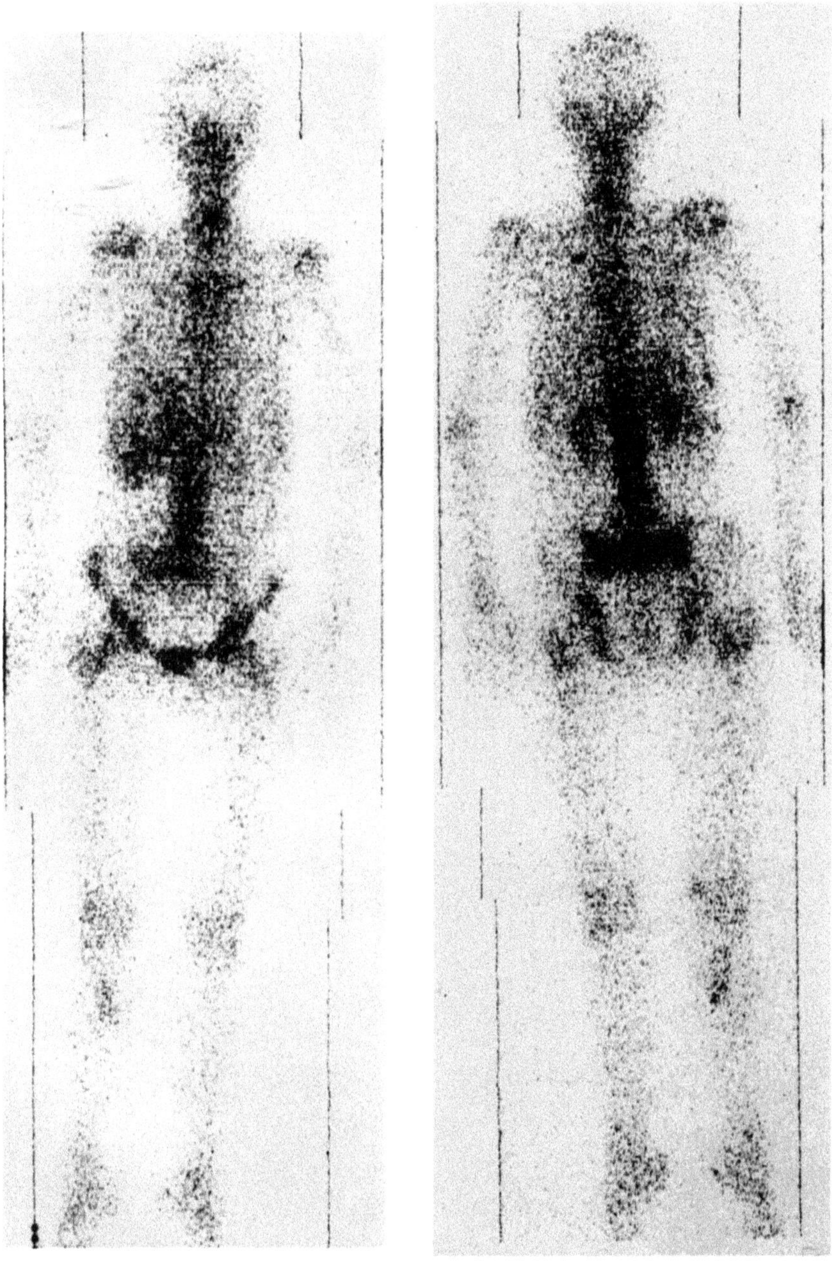

Fig. 6-12. Anterior and posterior 67Ga scan shows decreased uptake in the right lobe of the liver in a patient with marked hepatic failure. Multiple bony metastases are present. Note the renal route of excretion. Kidneys were free of tumor at autopsy.

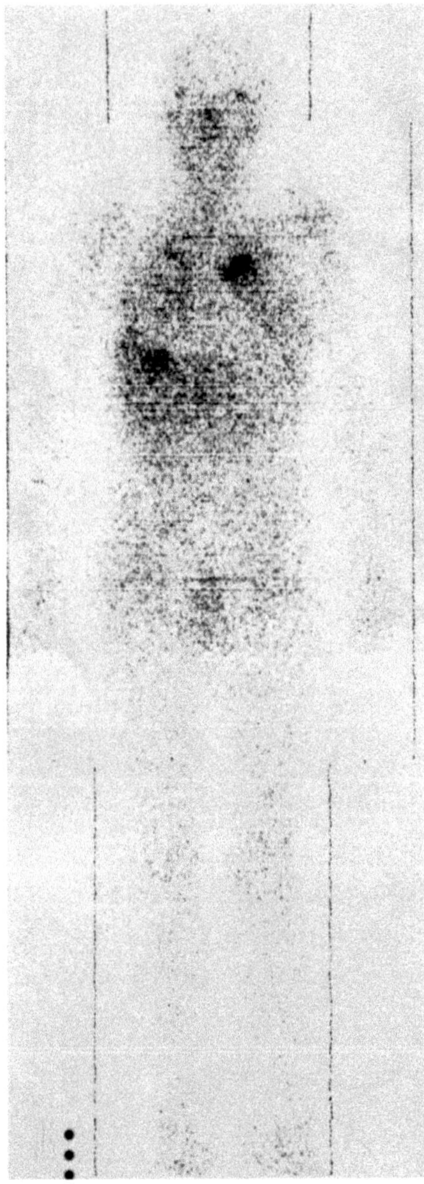

Fig. 6-13. Gallium-67 uptake in the right lower and left upper lung fields in a 65 year-old woman with a right radical mastectomy and pulmonary metastases. Gallium-67 abnormalities corresponded with large lung nodules. Liver biopsy was normal.

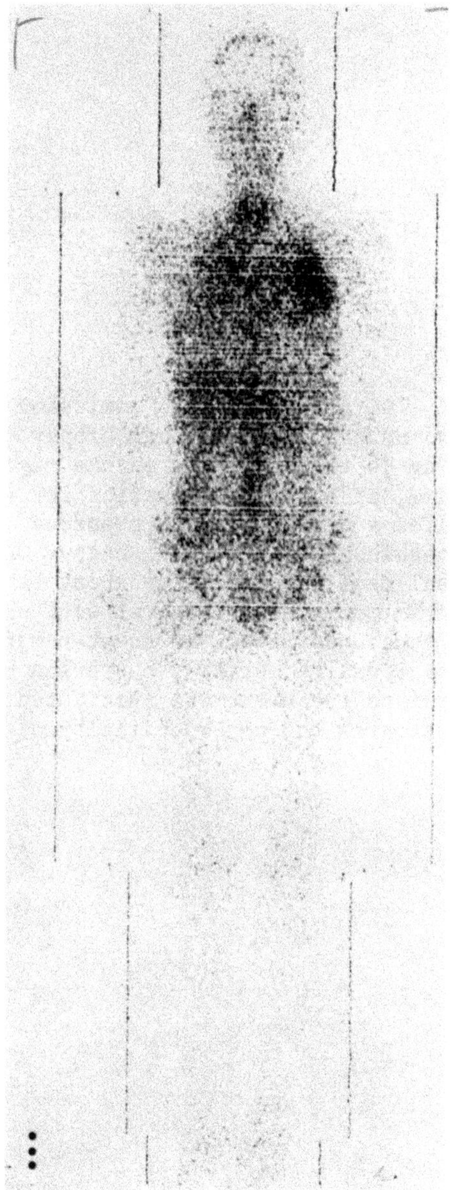

Fig. 6-14. Increased 67Ga uptake throughout both lungs accurately confirmed diffuse pulmonary metastases.

Fig. 6-15. Two years prior to admission this 38 year-old woman had an excisional biopsy for infiltrating ductal carcinoma in the right breast. At that time, abdominal exploration for a pelvic mass revealed a cystic papillary serous cystadenocarcinoma of the right ovary. A right paratracheal mass discovered on chest roentgenogram prompted a clinical work-up. Gallium-67 scan confirmed the chest tumor. Thoracotomy revealed metastatic ovarian carcinoma and appropriate treatment was instituted. This case demonstrates the non-specificity of 67Ga uptake.

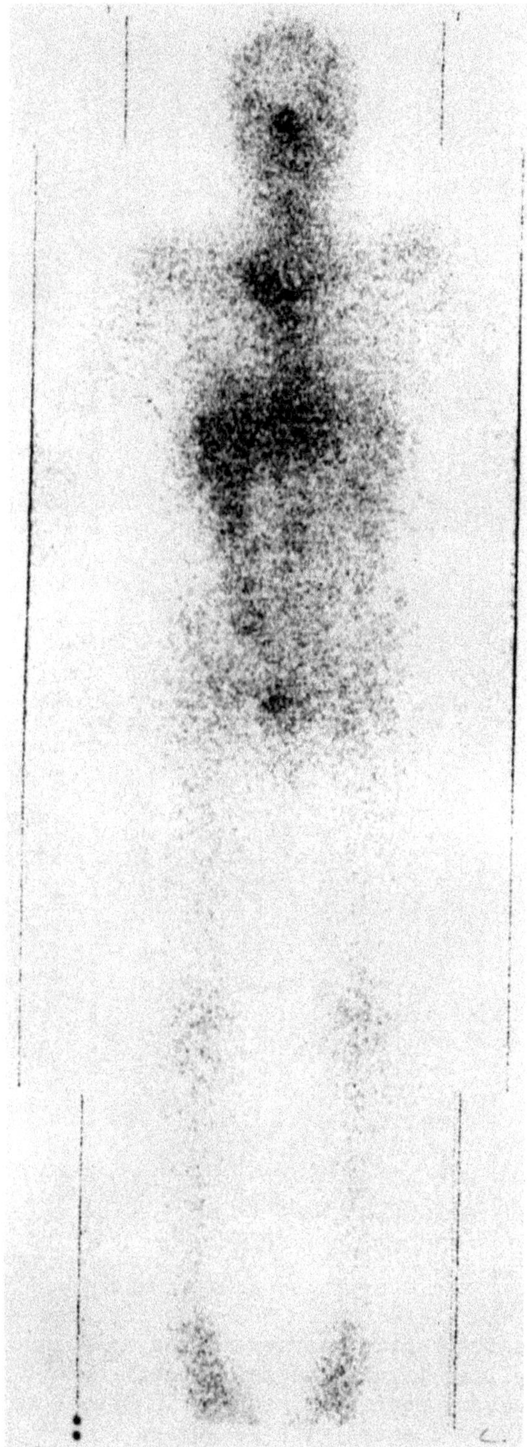

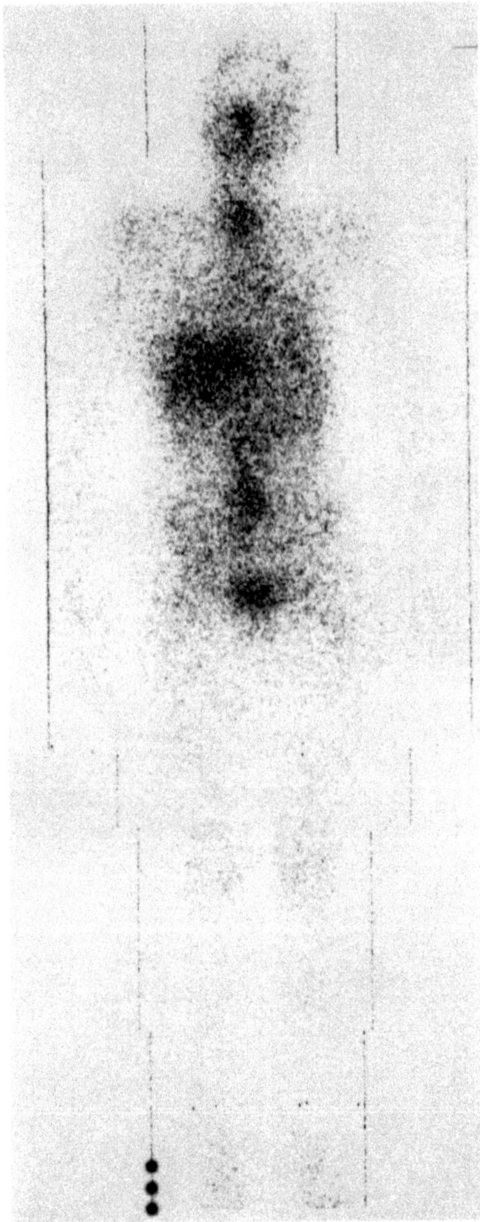

Fig. 6-16. Three years prior to admission this 55 year-old woman had a left radical mastectomy. Symptoms included at the time of this study were dysphagia, hoarseness and dyspnea on exertion. Gallium-67 localized in the thoracic inlet region. Biopsy at the time of tracheostomy confirmed metastatic breast carcinoma. (Abdominal activity cleared with laxatives.)

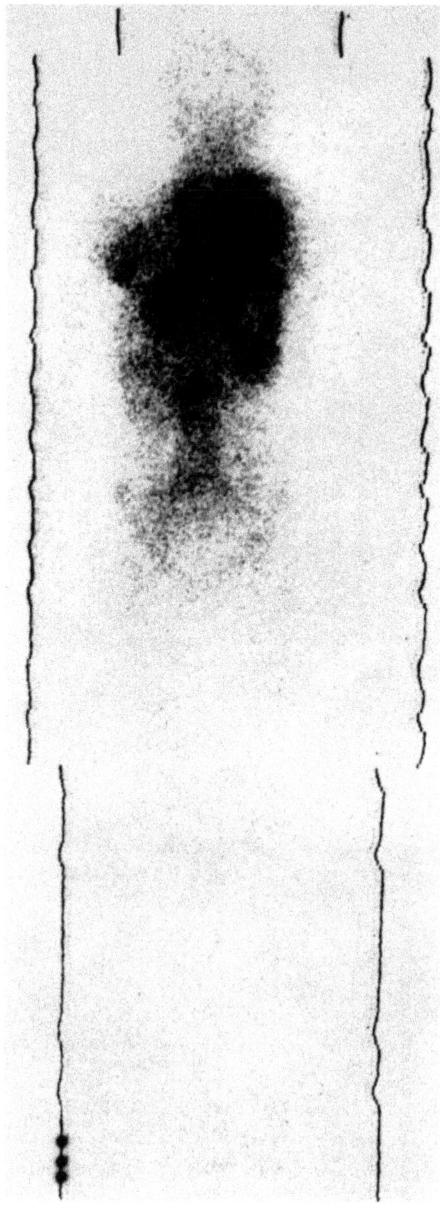

Fig. 6-17. Anterior scan of a 56 year-old woman with intense uptake in a massive, fixed, left breast tumor involving both chest walls and bilateral axillary regions.

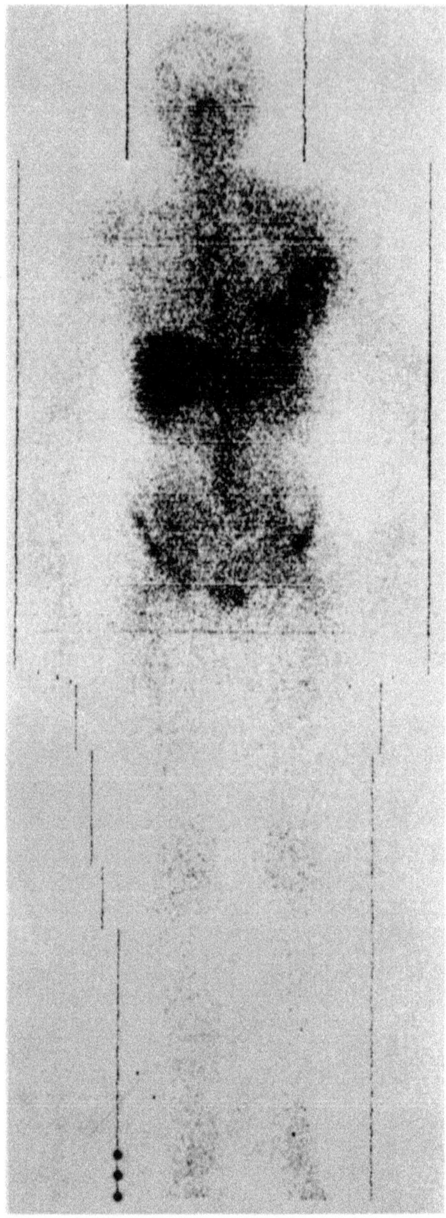

Fig. 6-18. Seven years after a right radical mastectomy this 53 year-old woman presented with disseminated metastases. There is 67Ga localization in the left breast, left axilla, and left supraclavicular nodes. Abnormal iliac activity represents bony metastases.

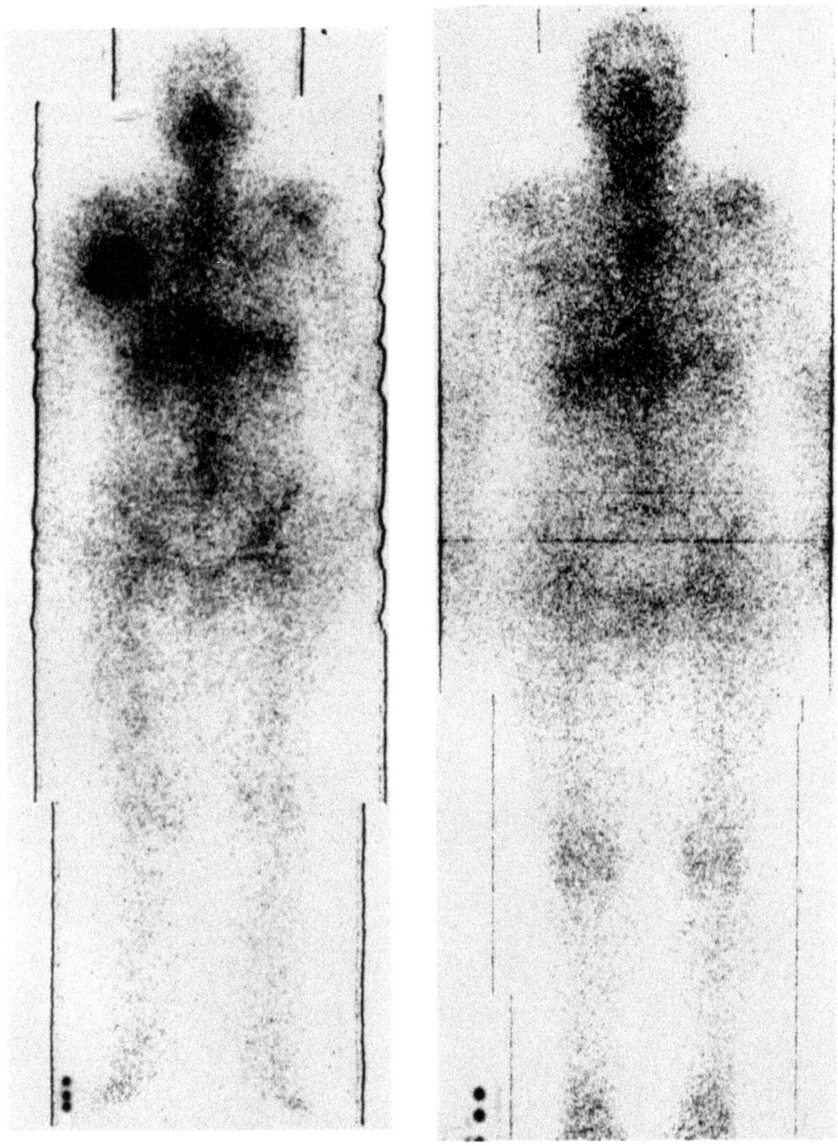

Fig. 6-19. A large inflammatory carcinoma of the right breast with intense 67Ga is seen in this study (left). After effective therapy the lesion improved clinically and 67Ga scan returned to normal (right).

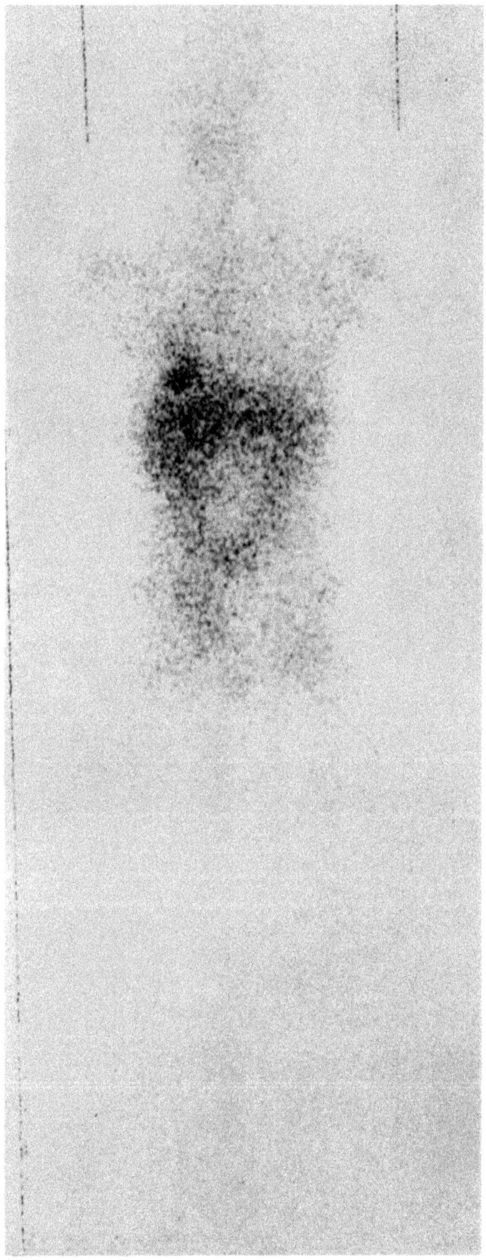

Fig. 6-20. Three weeks after surgery 67Ga localized in an infected mastectomy site, but failed to demonstrate known bony metastases.

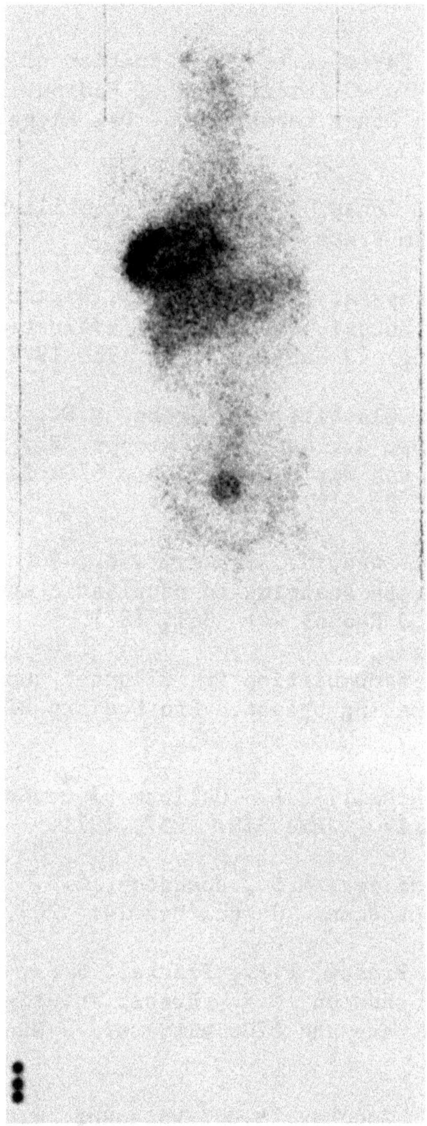

Fig. 6-21. Gallium-67 uptake throughout the right breast of this 35 year-old woman two months after left mastectomy. The patient was lactating in the post-operative period (prolactin levels were elevated). Persistent focal activity in the pelvis represents 67Ga uptake in an asymptomatic uterine fibroid confirmed at the time of oophorectomy.

References Chapter 6

1. Edwards, C.L., Hayes, R.L. Localization of tumors with radiosotopes. (In) Clinical Uses of Radionuclides: Critical Comparison with Other Techniques. Oak Ridge, Tennessee, 618, 1971.

2. Johnston, G.S., Jones, A.E. Atlas of Gallium 67 Scintigraphy. New York, Plenum Press, 1973.

3. Higasi, T., Nakayama, Y., Murata, A., Nakamure, K., Sugiyama, M., Kawaguchi, T., Suzuki, S. Clinical evaluation of 67Ga citrate scanning. J Nucl Med 13: 196, 1972.

4. Langhammer, H., Glaubitt, G., Grebe, S.F., Hampe, J.F., Haubold, U., Hor, G., Kaul, S., Keoppe, P., Koppenhagen, J., Roedler, H.D., van der Schoot, J.B. 67Ga for tumor scanning J Nucl Med 13: 25, 1972.

5. Lavender, J.P., Lowe, J., Barker, J.R., Burn, J.I., Chauhdri, M.A. Gallium 67 citrate scanning in neoplastic and inflammatory . lesions. Brit J Radiol 44: 361, 1971.

6. Fogh, J. 67Ga accumulation in malignant tumors and in the pre-lacting or lactating breast. Pro Soc Exp Biol Med 138: 1086, 1971.

7. Larson, S.M., Schall, G.L. Gallium 67 concentration in human breast milk. JAMA 218: 257, 1971.

8. Larson, S.M., Milder, M.S., Johnston, G.S. Interpretation of the 67Ga photoscan. J Nucl Med 14: 208, 1973.

9. Richman, S.D., Brodey, P.A., Frankel, R.S., de Moss, E.V., Tormey, D.C., Johnston, G.S. Breast scintigraphy with 99mTc pertechnetate and 67Ga citrate. J Nucl Med 16: 293, 1975.

10. Winchell, H.S., Sanchez, P.D., Watanabe, C.K., Hollander, L., Anger, H.O., McRae, J. Visualization of tumors in humans using 67Ga citrate and the Anger whole body scanner, scintillation camera and tomographic scanner. J Nucl Med 11: 459, 1970.

11. Harvey, W.C., Poduluff, D.A., Kopp, D.T. 67Gallium in 68 consecutive infection searches. J. Nucl. Med 16: 2, 1975.

12. Littenberg, R.L., Taketa, R.M., Alazraki, N., et al. Gallium 67 for localization of septic lesions. Ann Intern Med 79: 403, 1973.

CHAPTER 7

Radiologic Evaluation: Roentgenographic and Other Procedures

George S. Flinn, M.D., Robert S. Francis, M.D., Stanley M. Levenson, M.D.

Department of Radiology, Clinical Center
Department of Nuclear Medicine, Clinical Center
National Institutes of Health
Bethesda, Maryland

The contribution of diagnostic radiology in the initial detection and follow-up of patients with carcinoma of the breast (1) is well accepted. Techniques and procedures used in the radiographic evaluation of patients with suspected or established carcinoma of the breast have become routine diagnostic methods in this disease. Thermography and ultrasonography are being evaluated as aids in breast cancer diagnosis in many radiology departments. A common sequence of application of these methods includes:

Breast Evaluation

Mammography and Xeroradiography: Conventional film mammography (2,3,4) and xeroradiography (5) are the most reliable studies in the evaluation of suspicious breast masses (Figs. 7-1, 7-2, 7-3). However, the role of mammography in large-scale screening of asymptomatic patients has yet to be defined. Only after long-term prospective surveys have provided adequate data can valid recommendations be made on the optimum type and frequency of x-ray examination and patient selection.

Until recently, a usual policy has been to perform both conventional low killivolt (KV), high MAS (milliampsec) non-screen film mammograms along with xeroradiographs during the initial evaluation of a patient with a breast tumor. In follow-up studies, only mammograms were utilized. Presently, however, in an effort to reduce the patient radiation dose (6) and simplify the procedure, xeroradiography is used exclusively. This is accomplished with a 1.0 mm focal spot tungsten tube interfaced to a single phase, full wave rectified generator and inherent aluminum filtration. Tube-film distance is 30-36 inches. Exposure factors in the positive mode are 33-42 KV at 400-450 MAS. Craniocaudad and mediolateral views are routinely obtained. The axilla is usually well visualized on the mediolateral view, obviating additional axillary images. Compression on the craniocaudad view is obtained by inserting an inflated balloon into the "mouth" of a long cone. The balloon is firm and exerts adequate pressure on the breast without causing discomfort. Conventional mammography is rarely used, as only occasional cases have been seen where microcalcifications were more easily visualized on mammograms than on xeroradiographs.

The indications for mammography are quite broad with the aim being to differentiate a benign breast process from malignant disease. The following are indications for mammography:

1. Patients presenting with breast masses, pain or nipple discharge.
2. The baseline examination of the "lumpy" breast.
3. Large breasts in patients with a new breast complaint (large breasts can prevent palpation of a cancer easily seen on mammograms).
4. A screening or localizing procedure prior to breast biopsy.
5. Confirmation of clinical breast cancer.
6. Evaluation of the remaining breast for carcinoma after mastectomy, (This high risk group of patients comprises a large percentage of patients with mammograms at our institution.
7. Family history of breast carcinoma. These patients have a 2-3 fold increased incidence of breast carcinoma.
8. Unknown primary cancer and metastases in an adult female.

Thermography: Thermography is another technique for breast examination (7,8,9,10). The thermogram registers the heat pattern of the breast via a monitor sensitive to infra-red radiation. The increased metabolic rate of tumors causes increased heat production resulting in an abnormal thermal pattern. Thermograms are easily performed but difficult to interpret, and have a significant false-positive rate of 15-20%. The inexact nature of the technique precludes its use as a single mass screening procedure. The thermogram is always used in conjunction with physical exam. When there is an abnormal thermogram, supplemental mammography should be obtained prior to breast biopsy.

Ultrasonography: Ultrasonographic examination of the breast

(11,12,13,14,15) is being evaluated as a screening procedure by many investigators, but is neither generally available, nor widely accepted. Its use in the examination of a breast mass is considered quite accurate in differentiating between cystic (Figs. 7-4) and solid breast lesions. The most accurate mode of ultrasound scanning for small lesions is the A-scan, although the B-scan is now being utilized with both cystic and solid lesions which are easily identified if the lesion is palpable. With improvements in instrumentation and further physician experience, ultrasonography appears to be a promising modality in screening for breast disease.

Detection of Metastases

Metastatic Survey: Because of the frequency of skeletal involvement, plain film radiographs of the axial and appendicular skeleton are used in conjunction with bone scans for the initial detection of bony metastases (16,17,18,19,20,21). The bone scan has been invaluable in isolating specific areas for special tomographic evaluation. Chapter 5 presents and describes the value of bone scintigraphy in patients with breast carcinoma.

The skeletal survey, the frequency of which is being re-evaluated in this patient population, is performed in the following manner. The routine metastatic survey includes AP and lateral projections of the lumbar and thoracic spine, lateral cervical spine, 3-view skull, AP pelvis including proximal femurs (Fig. 7-5A,B,C), PA and lateral chest, AP views of upper and lower extremities, and any indicated projections of symptomatic regions (Fig. 7-6). Rib detail views have been especially helpful in conjunction with suspicious bone scans. The bone survey has been useful in differentiating areas of degenerative or benign bone disease in the presence of an abnormal bone scan. Its particular value appears to be in the follow-up of skeletal metastases detected by skeletal scintigraphy (Fig. 7-7A,B,C,D,E,) and in determining response to chemotherapy.

Tomography: Tomographic examination of suspicious areas seen on plain films, e.g., the spine, in which the extent of involvement needs further definition, has become standard procedure. It is also quite common to perform tomography on the cervicothoracic junction, sacrum, sternum and other sites, which though not necessarily suspicious, are otherwise difficult to adequately define.

Full-lung tomography warrants significant consideration. A review of all full-lung tomograms performed over a one year period in our department demonstrated several cases of positive tomograms with metastatic nodules. Corresponding radiographs were normal. Full-lung tomography utilizing linear sweep in 1 cm. sections has been of value in the initial evaluation and follow-up of metastatic lung disease in breast carcinoma patients (Fig. 7-8A,B).

Ultrasonography: Ultrasound examination of the liver (22,23,24,25,26,27) using conventional bistable equipment is much less sensitive than liver scintigraphy in the evaluation of hepatic metastases (Fig. 7-9). Ultrasound can differentiate between cystic and solid lesions in the liver, and this may well evolve to be the prime value of the hepatic ultrasound examination. Another potential use of this modality is the determination of temporal size changes in metastatic liver lesions; some suggest that ultrasound will supplant the routine liver scan for this purpose in the future. In addition, focal "cold" areas noted on 99mTc sulfur colloid liver scan may be evaluated by ultrasound examination. Intrahepatic gallbladder and enlarged portal vein might be differentiated from metastases by ultrasonography. At present,hepatic ultrasonography isdifficult because of the interference of ribs when imaging the liver.

Special Procedures: The need for angiography occasionally arises in the evaluation of metastatic disease. Carotid angiography in patients with neurologic manifestations suggesting intracerebral metastases can be helpful when the brain scan is positive or equivocal. The availability of computerized axial tomography (C.A.T.) for the evaluation of brain lesions may further modify the approach to those patients now requiring carotid angiography.

Abdominal angiography is rarely necessary for evaluation of visceral metastases. In the occasional patient with gastrointestinal hemorrhage secondary to metastases or chemotherapy, visceral angiography is helpful in localizing the site of bleeding. Hemorrhaging can hopefully then be controlled by the selective infusion of vasopressors or selective embolization of the bleeding site.

Myelography is often used to diagnose and localize the site of spinal metastases. These are usually extradural deposits having spread contiguously from bony metastases. The contrast material is usually left in the subarachnoid space after the procedure to allow radiographic visualization of tumor response to therapy.

In summary, an overview of the radiographic, thermographic, and ultrasonographic methods of evaluating patients with suspected or proven breast carcinoma has been presented. No attempt has been made to list all the possible radiographic modalities or to dogmatically recommend their specific use. The ramifications of whole-body C.A.T. scanning systems will certainly change the future application of diagnostic radiology with hopeful benefit for patients with breast carcinoma.

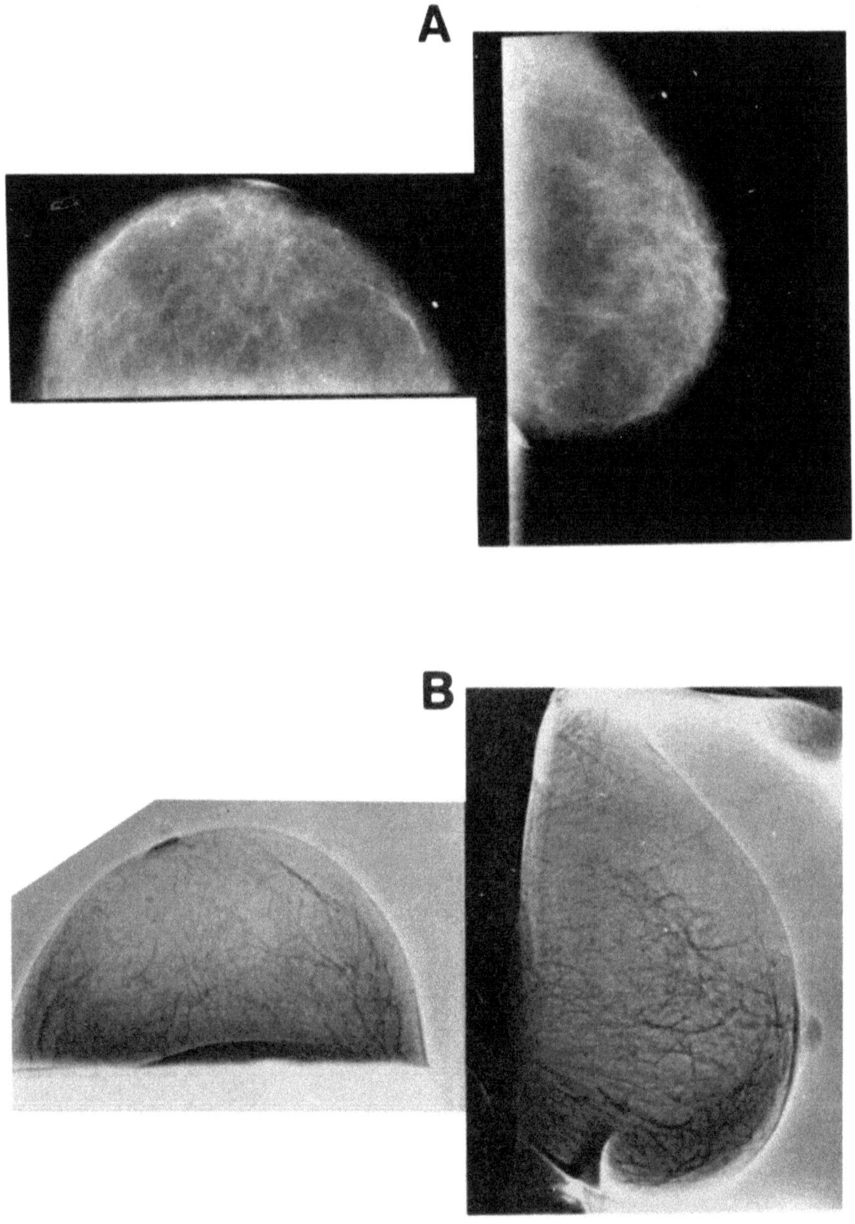

Fig. 7-1. Following radical mastectomy this 64 year old woman had mammographic (A) and xeroradiographic (B) examinations of her right breast. Minimal atrophic changes are seen in an otherwise unremarkable breast. (Note: For Figs. 7-1, 7-2, and 7-3, craniocaudad view appears on left and lateral view adjacent on right).

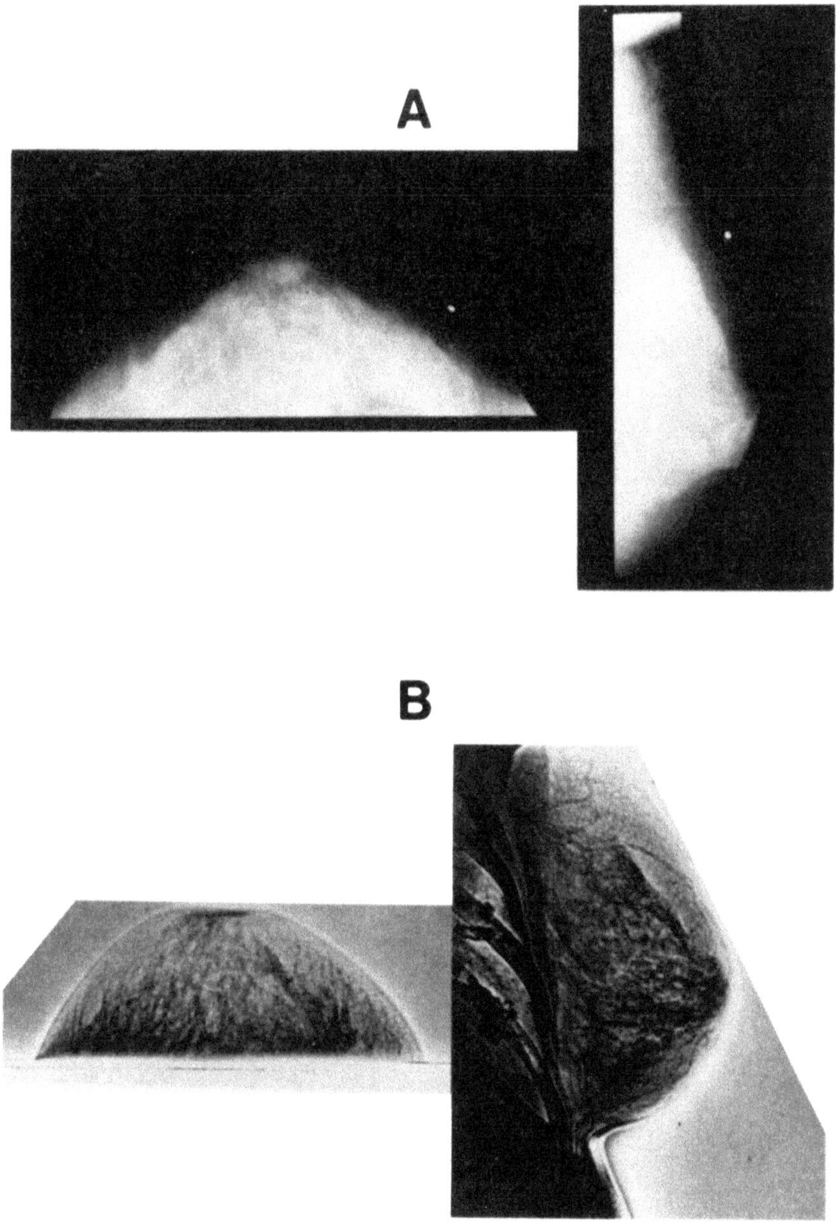

Fig. 7-2. Mammogram (A) and xeroradiogram (B) demonstrate fibrous dysplasia in the remaining right breast of this 65 year old woman.

A

B

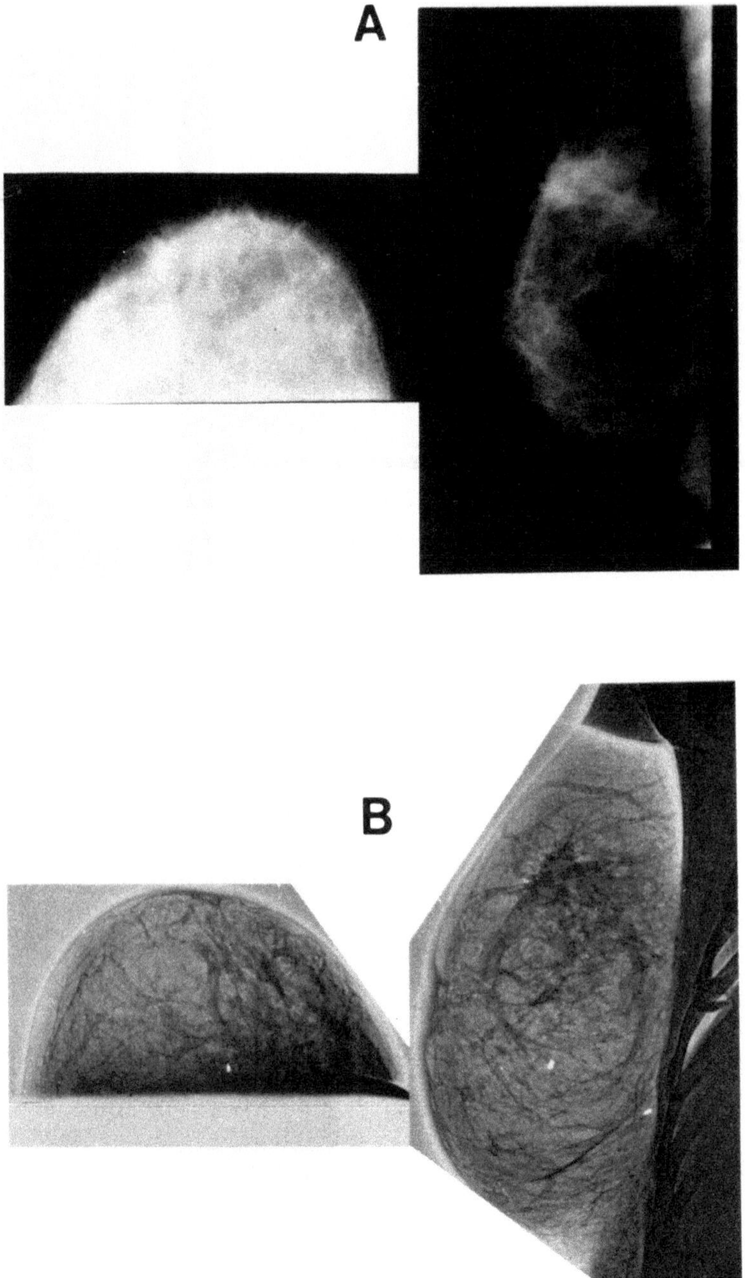

Fig. 7-3. A primary breast carcinoma is seen in the upper outer quadrant of this 45 year old woman's left breast. It is well-demarcated both mammographically (A) and xeroradiographically (B). (Note: Craniocaudad view in 7-3B is mirror image; lesion therefore appears medial instead of lateral).

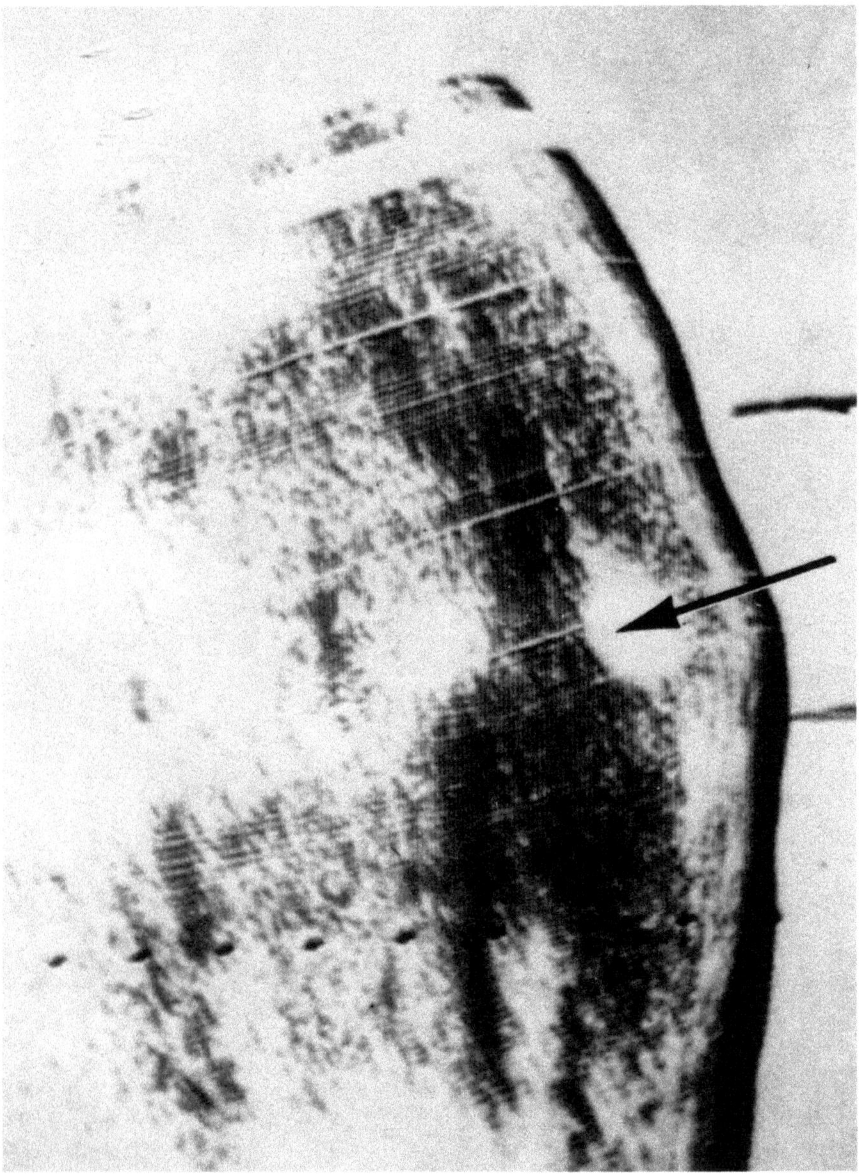

Fig. 7-4. Ultrasound image of right breast: Longitudinal sonogram 1cm. lateral to the nipple demonstrates cystic disease (arrow).

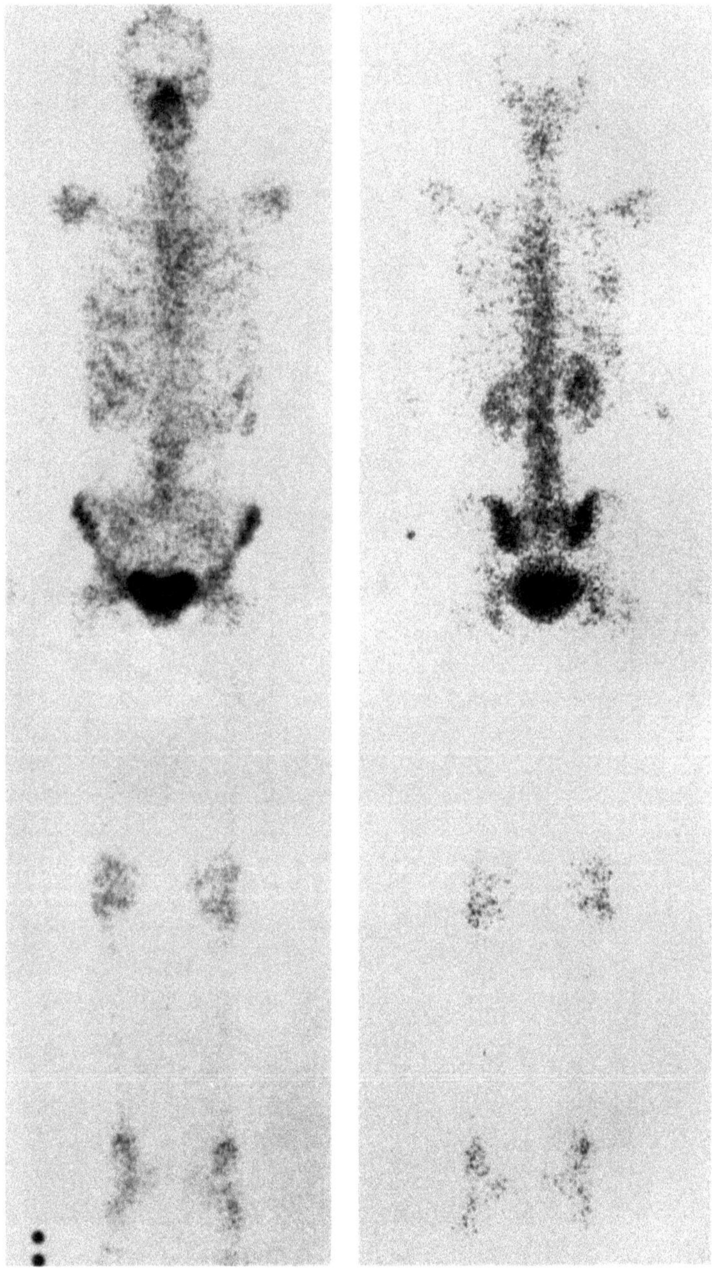

Fig. 7-5A. Serial bone scans over a seven month interval were similar to this, and failed to reveal any definite bony pelvic asymmetries.

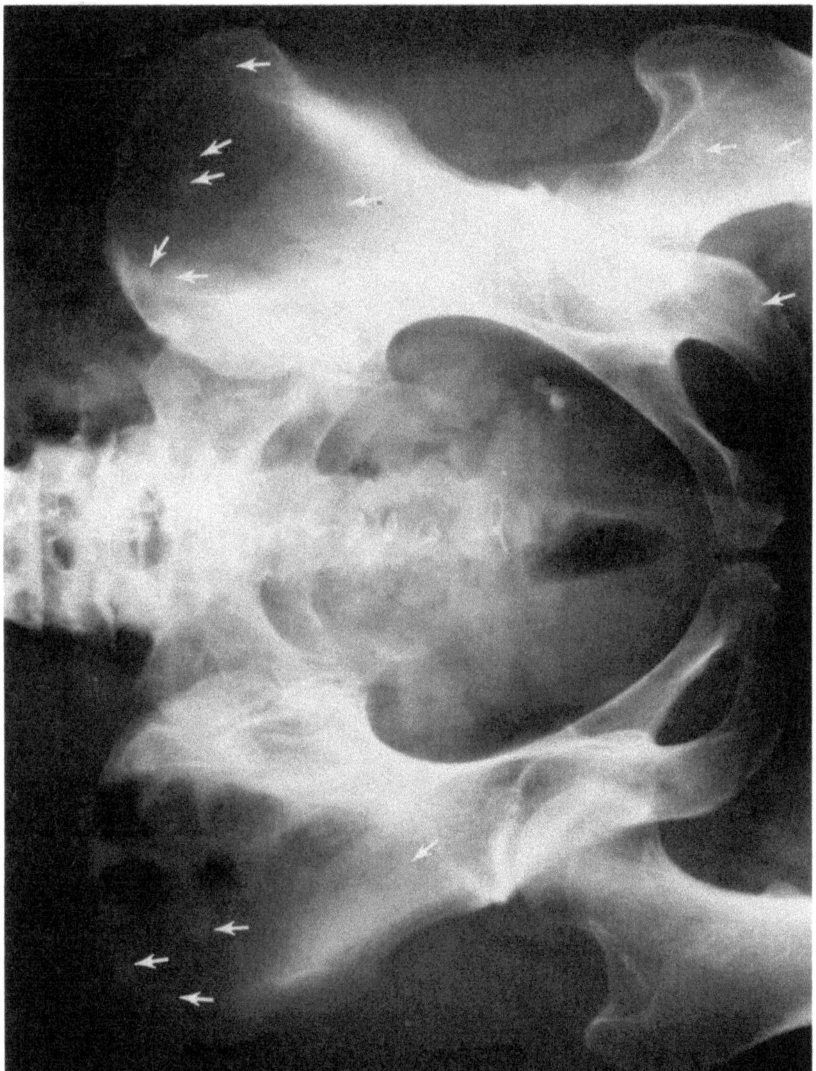

Fig. 7-5B. Pelvic roentgenogram at the onset of this period demonstrates multiple osteoblastic metastases involving the pelvis and proximal femur.

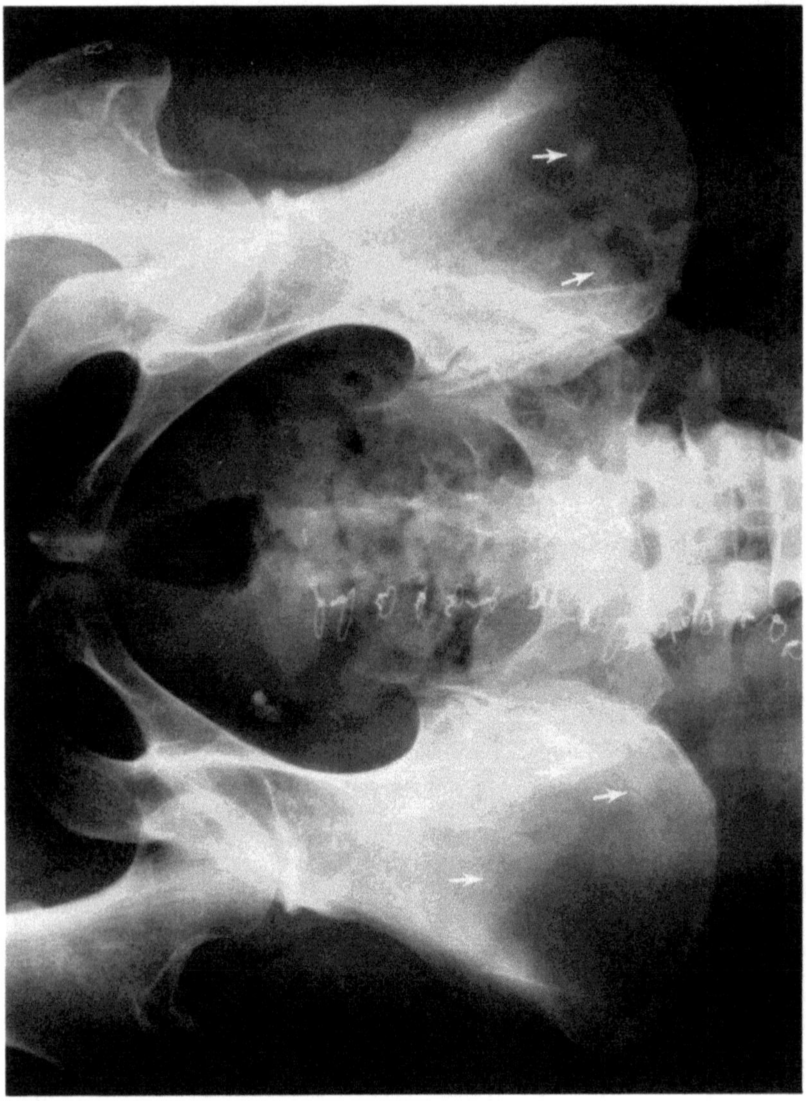

Fig. 7-5C. Despite the persistent absence of pelvic bone scan findings, obvious radiographic improvement is noted. Osteoblastic metastases, particularly in this location using the whole-body 5:1 reduction images, may cause false negative interpretations. Roentgenographic follow-up was clearly superior in this situation.

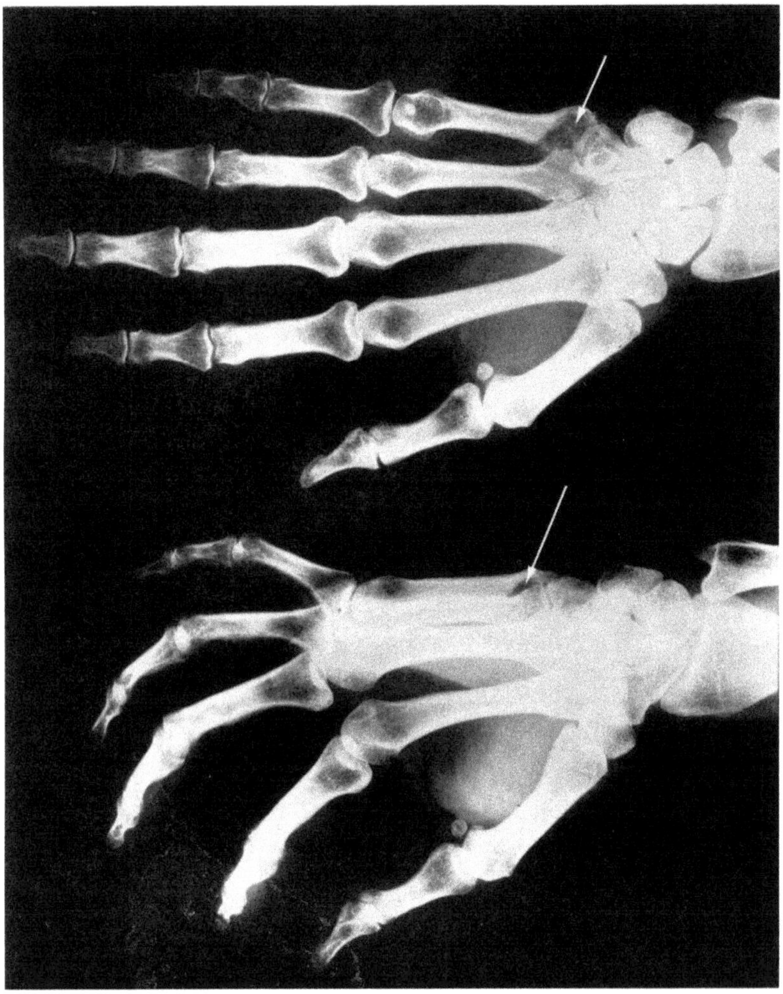

Fig. 7-6. Lytic metastasis to proximal right 5th metacarpal. Routine whole-body rectilinear scanning for bony metastases distal to the humerus has been unrewarding. Radiographic techniques may be more sensitive in detecting these uncommon sites. In the presence of localized bone pain, special camera views are advisable.

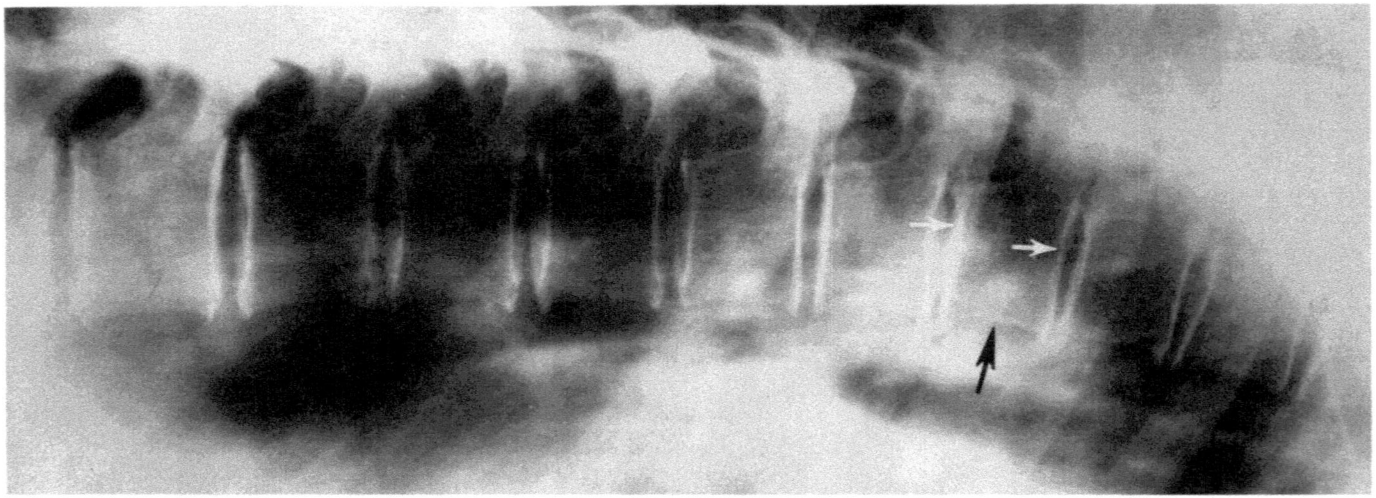

Fig. 7-7A. Metastatic bone disease can be more accurately assessed roentgenographically, following its initial detection by bone scan. Radiograph of the dorsal spine reveals only minimal degenerative changes.

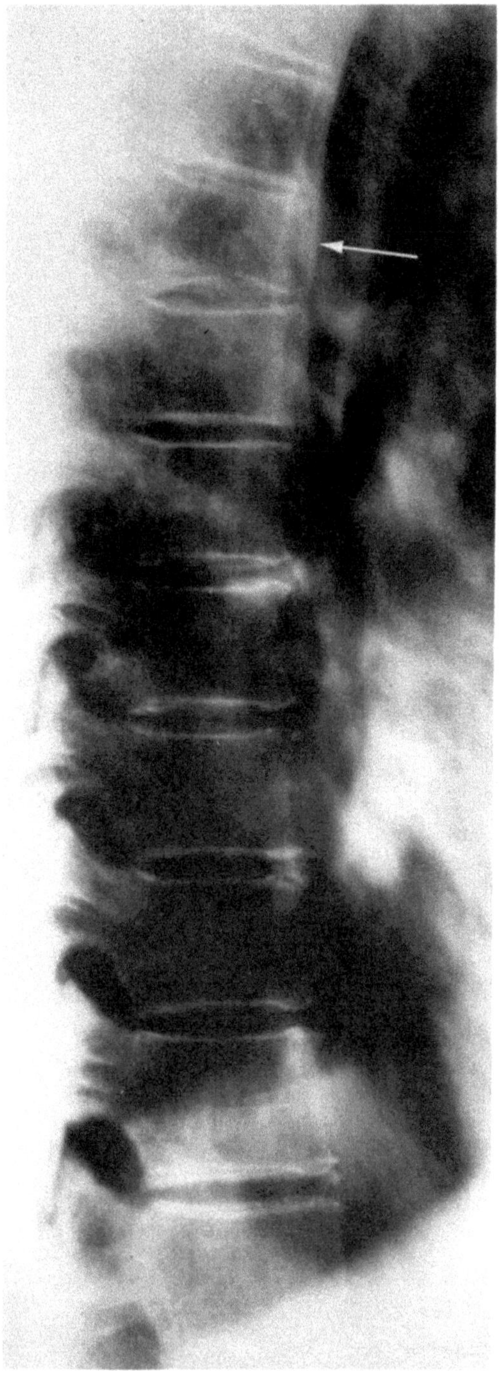

Fig. 7-7B. Three months following the first radiograph infraction of the superior and inferior end plates of T-5 is noted.

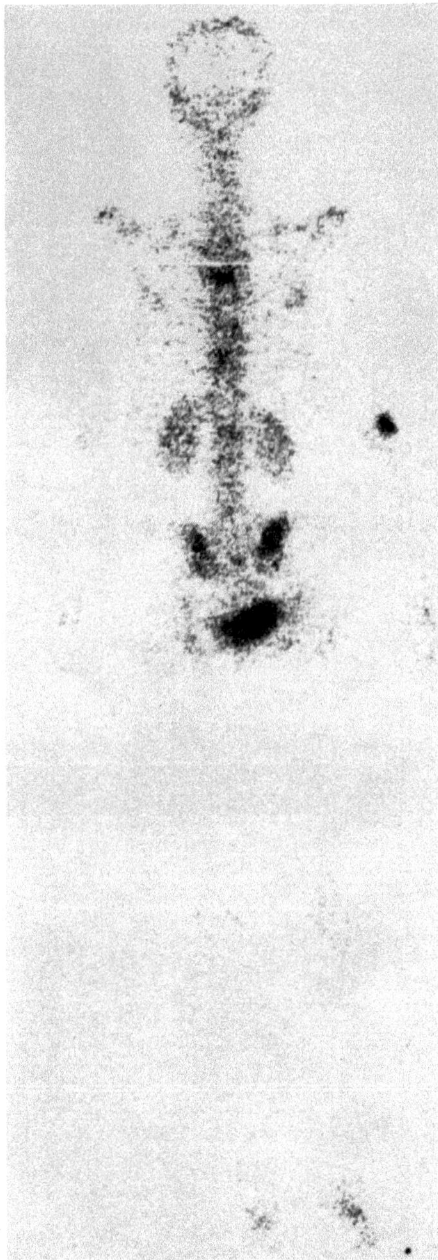

Fig. 7-7C. Posterior bone scan at the time of the Fig. 7-7B radiograph confirms this lesion and reveals additional suspicious tracer increases at T10-11, L-2 and the right sacroiliac joint.

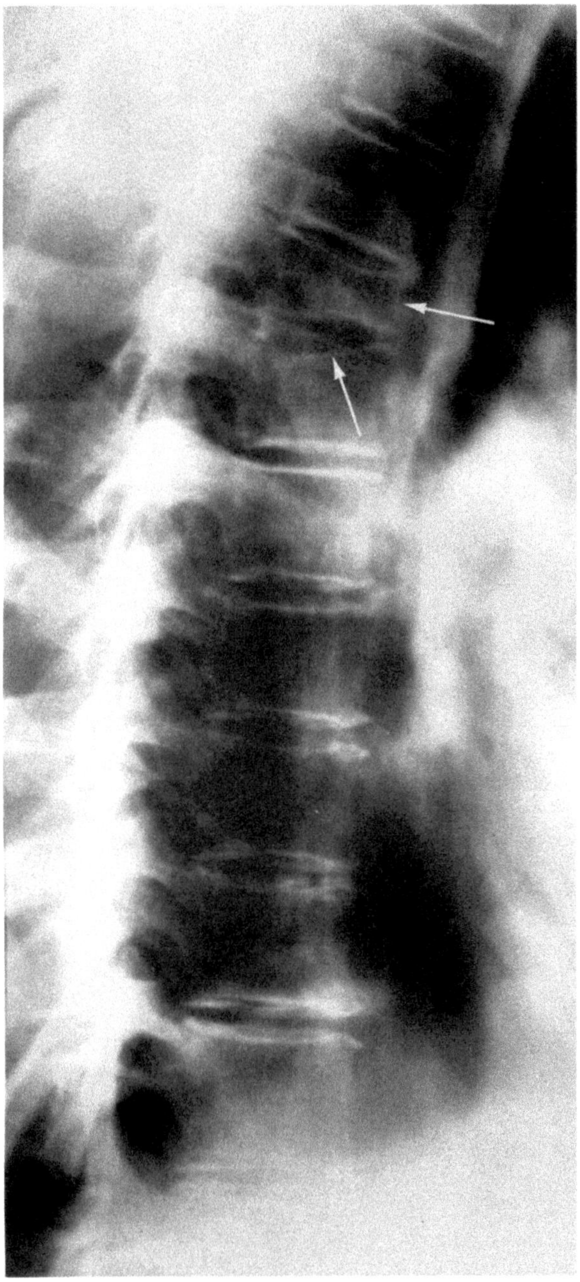

Fig. 7-7D. Follow-up radiograph five months later demonstrates disease progression with compression fracture of T-5 and depression of the T-6 superior end-plate.

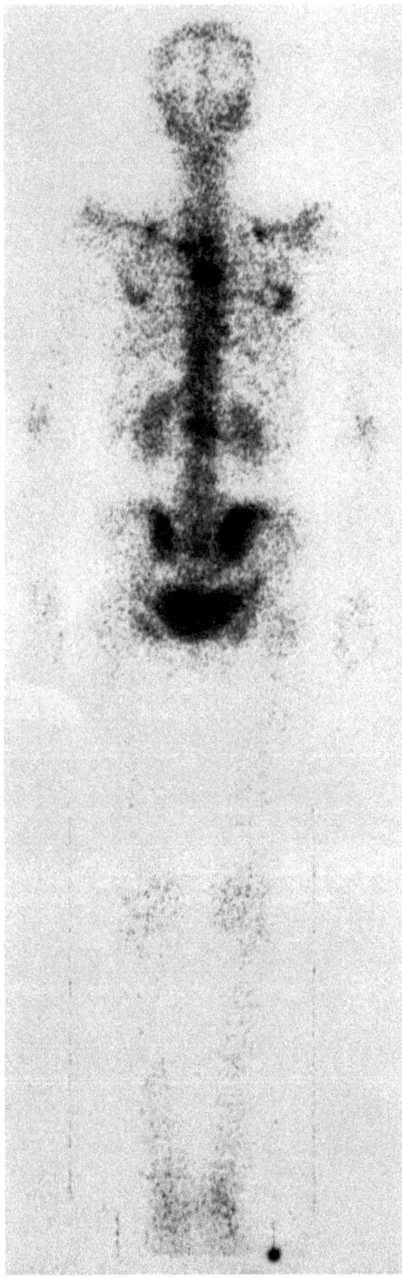

Fig. 7-7E. The bone scan, while more sensitive for detecting new metastatic disease, provides no further definition of disease progression at T5-6.

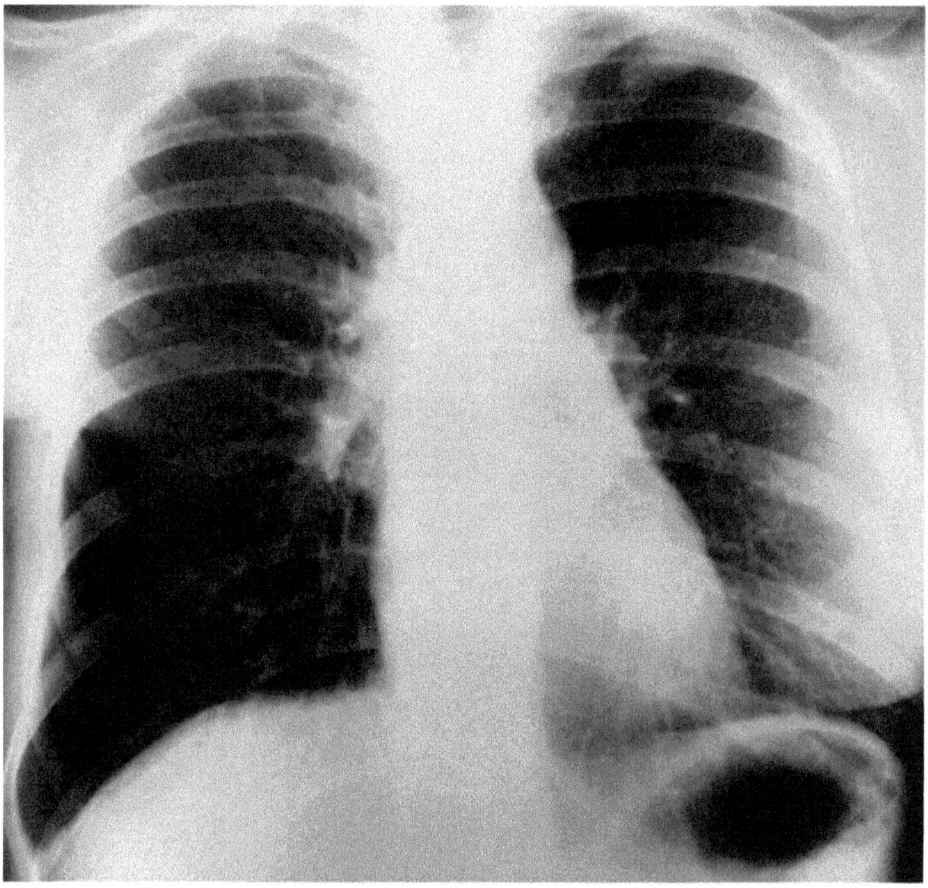

Fig. 7-8A. Chest radiograph in this post-right mastectomy patient demonstrated minimal fullness in the right hilum.

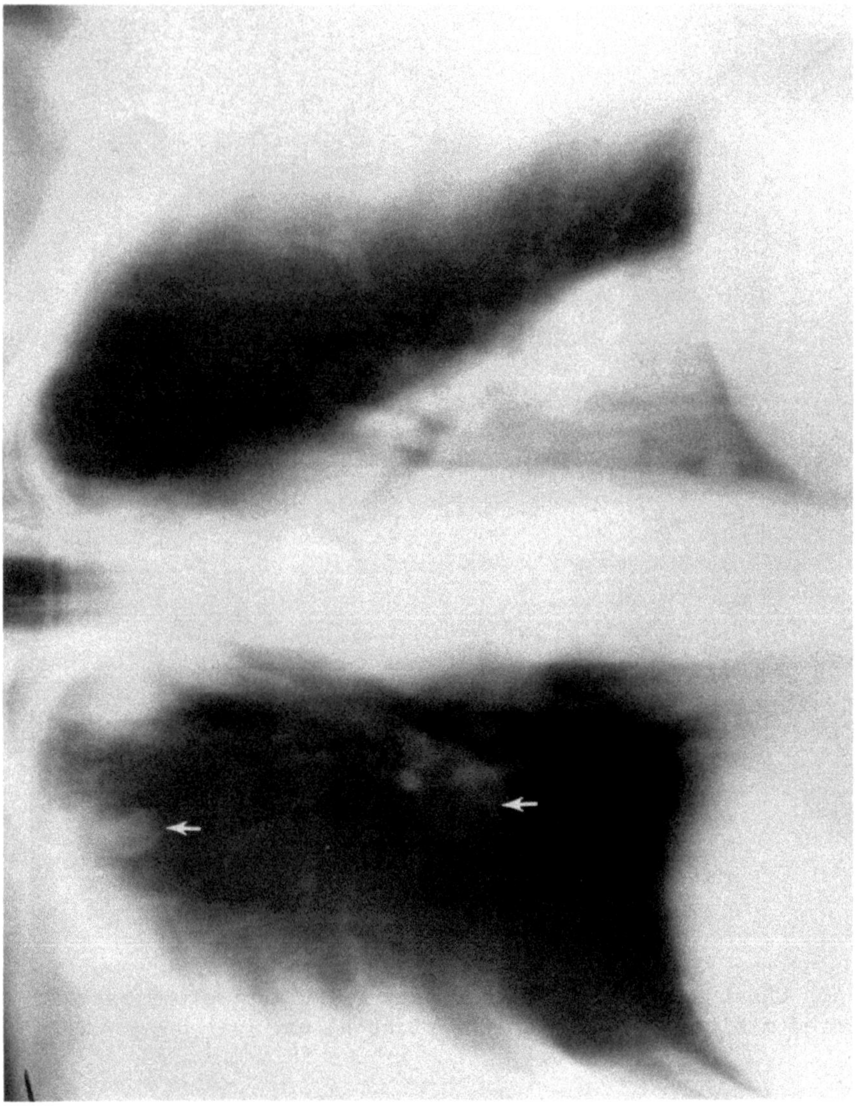

Fig. 7-8B. Full-lung tomography revealed a definite right hilar mass, in addition to an unsuspected right apical pulmonary metastasis. The value of tomography in the detection of secondary pulmonary involvement is apparent.

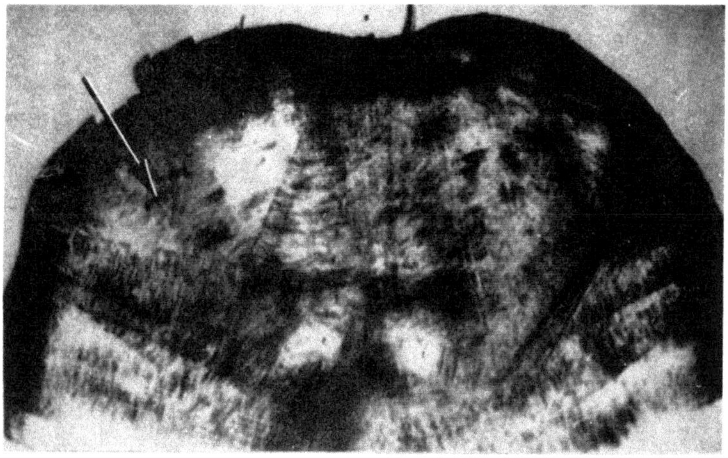

A

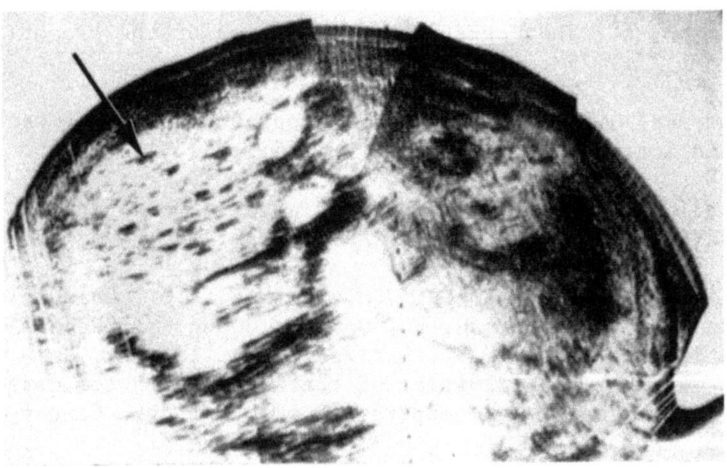

B

Fig. 7-9. Ultrasound images of the liver: Transverse sections 2 cms. beneath the xyphoid demonstrate the difficulty in hepatic evaluation with this technique. Note the similarity of the echo pattern in (A) hepatic metastases and (B) areas of post-inflammatory focal fibrosis. Arrow in right lobe identifies one of many abnormal areas.

References Chapter 7

1. Gershon-Cohen, J. Imperative changes in detection method for breast cancer. So Med J 64: 387, 1971.

2. Leger, J-L., Naimark, A.P., Beique, R.A., McFarlane, D.V., Miller, S., Miller, A.B. Report of the "Ad Hoc" committee on mammography. J Canad Assn Radiol 25: 3, 1974.

3. Egan, R.L. Mammography and breast disease. Baltimore, Md. Williams and Wilkins, 1970.

4. Egan, R.L. Mammography. 2nd Ed. Springfield, Ill., Charles C. Thomas, 1972

5. Wolfe, J.N. Xeroradiography of the breast. Springfield, Ill., Charles C. Thomas, 1972.

6. Palmer, R.C., Egan, R.L., Tanner, B.K., Barnette, P.A. Absorbed dose in mammography using tungsten and molybdenum target tubes. Radiology 101: 697, 1971.

7. Dodd., G.D., Wallace, J.D., Freundlich, I.M., Marsh, L., Zermino, A. Thermography and carcinoma of the breast. Cancer 23: 797, 1969.

8. Haberman, J.D. The role of thermography in breast cancer detection. Proc Natl Cancer Conf 6: 157, 1970.

9. Isard, H.J. Breast thermography after 4 years and 10,000 studies. Amer J Roentgenol Radium Ther Nucl Med 115: 811, 1972.

10. Lilienfeld, A.M., Barnes, J.M., Barnes, R.B., Brasfield, R., Connell, J.F., Diamond, E., Gershon-Cohen, J., Haberman, J., Isard, H.J., Lane, W.Z., Lattes, R., Miller, J., Seaman, W., Sherman, R. An evaluation of thermography in the detection of breast cancer: A cooperative pilot study. Cancer 24: 1206, 1969.

11. Damascelli, B., Fossati, F., Livraghi, T., Severini, A. B-scan ultrasound exploration of neoplastic disease. Amer J Roentgenol Radium Ther Nucl Med, 105: 428, 1969.

12. DeLand, F. Modified technique of ultrasonography for detection and differential diagnosis of breast lesions. Amer J Roentgenol Radium Ther Nucl Med 105: 446, 1969.

13. Jellins, J., Kossoff, G., Buddee, F.W., Reeve, T.S. Ultrasonic visualization of the breast. Med J Aust 1: 305, 1971.

14. Wells, P.N.T., Evans, K.T. An immersion scanner for two-dimensional ultrasonic examination of the human breast. Ultrasonics 6: 220, 1968.

15. Kossoff, G., Fry, E.K., Jellins, J. Average velocity of ultrasound in the human female breast. J Acoust Soc Amer 53: 1730, 1973.

16. Abrams, H.L., Spiro, L.R., Goldstein, N. Metastasis in carcinoma. Analysis of 1,000 autopsied cases. Cancer 3: 74, 1950.

17. Carnett, J.B., Howell, J.C. Bone metastases in cancer of the breast. Ann Surg 91: 811, 1930.

18. Freid, J.R., Goldberg, H. Frequency, clinical course and treatment of metastases from cancer of the breast. Amer J Roentgenol Radium Ther Nucl Med 50: 499, 1943.

19. Lenz, M., Freid, J.R. Metastases to skeleton , brain and spinal cord from carcinoma of the breast and the effect of radiotherapy. Ann Surg 93: 278. 1931.

20. Warren, S., Witham, E.M. Studies on tumor metastases: The distribution of metastases in cancer of the breast. Surg Gyn Obstet 57: 81, 1933.

21. Turner, J.W., Jaffe, H.L. Metastatic neoplasms; A clinical and roentgenological study of involvement of skeleton and lungs. Amer J Roentgenol Radium Ther Nucl Med 43: 479, 1940.

22. Rasmussen, S.N., Holm, H.H., Kristensen, J.K., Pedersen, J.F., Hancke, S. Ultrasound in the diagnosis of liver disease. J Clin Ultrasound 1: 220, 1973.

23. McCarthy, C.F., Davies, E., Wells, P.N., Ross, F.G., Follett, D.H., Muir, K.M., Read, A.E. A comparison of ultrasonic and isotopic scanning in the diagnosis of liver disease. Brit J Rad 43: 100, 1970.

24. McCarthy, C.F., Read, A.E., Ross, F.G.M., Wells, P.N.T. Ultrasonic scanning of the liver. Quart J Med 35: 517, 1967.

25. Damascelli, B., Bonadonna, G., Roncoroni, L., Uslenghi, C., Veronesi, V. Two-dimensional ultrasounds in liver diseases. JAMA 204: 963, 1968.

26. Leyton, B., Halpen, S., Leopold., G., Hagen, S. Correlation of ultrasound and colloid scintiscan studies of the normal and diseased liver. J Nucl Med 14: 27, 1973.

27. Taylor, K.J.W., Carpenter, D.A., McCready, V.R. Grey scale echography in the diagnosis of intrahepatic disease. J Clin Ultrasound 1: 284, 1973.

INDEX

MIX
Papier aus verantwortungsvollen Quellen
Paper from responsible sources
FSC® C105338

If you have any concerns about our products,
you can contact us on
ProductSafety@springernature.com

In case Publisher is established outside the EU,
the EU authorized representative is:
Springer Nature Customer Service Center GmbH
Europaplatz 3, 69115 Heidelberg, Germany

Printed by Libri Plureos GmbH
in Hamburg, Germany